PLYOMETRICS

FOR ATHLETES AT ALL LEVELS

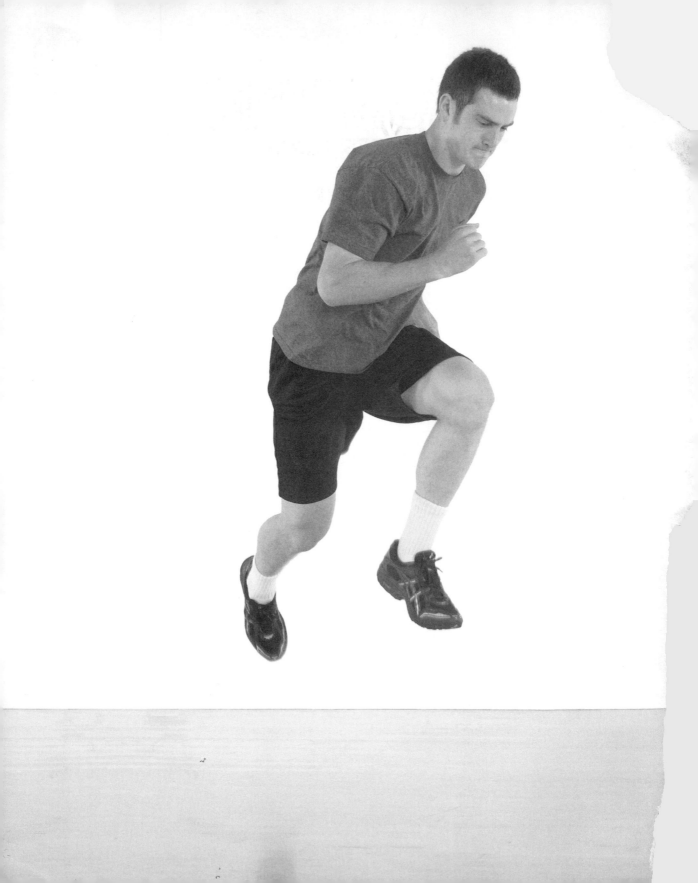

PLYOMETRICS

FOR ATHLETES AT ALL LEVELS

Exercises for Explosive Speed and Power

NEAL PIRE

photography by **Andy Mogg**

Ulysses Press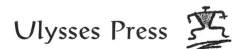

Published in the United States by Ulysses Press
                              P.O. Box 3440
                              Berkeley, CA 94703
                              www.ulyssespress.com

ISBN10: 1-56975-559-0
ISBN13: 978-1-56975-559-4
Library of Congress Control Number 2006903815

Printed in Canada by Webcom

10 9 8 7 6 5 4 3 2

Editorial/Production	Lily Chou, Claire Chun, Matt Orendorff, Steven Zah Schwartz
Index	Sayre Van Young
Cover design	Matt Orendorff
Interior photographs	Andy Mogg except on pages 9, 33, 35, 37, 41, 43, 45, 47, 49, 51, 53, 55, 57, 59, 61, 63, 65, 67, 69 © photos.com
Cover photographs	*front:* © Andy Mogg (male model), © photos.com (basketball, tennis ball, soccer ball, volleyball) © comstock.com (football); *back:* © photos.com
Models	Vanessa Alvarez, Samuel Denton-Schneider, Neal Pire

Distributed by Publishers Group West

Please Note
This book has been written and published strictly for informational purposes, and in no way should be used as a substitute for consultation with health care professionals. You should not consider educational material herein to be the practice of medicine or to replace consultation with a physician or other medical practitioner. The author and publisher are providing you with information in this work so that you can have the knowledge and can choose, at your own risk, to act on that knowledge. The author and publisher also urge all readers to be aware of their health status and to consult health care professionals before beginning any health program.

table of contents

6

part one:

jumping
out of
the fire

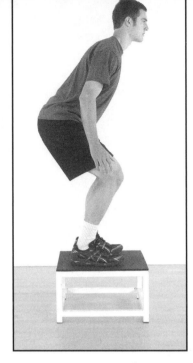

plyometrics: an overview

Plyometrics has quickly become one of the most popular sports-training methods on the planet. Research has shown it to be an effective way to use your body's own anatomical and physiological systems to improve athletic performance.

In an age when shaving a tenth of a second off your 40 can be the deciding factor in getting an athletic scholarship to a Division I school or corporate firm partnership is based on your success on the golf course, it's imperative that you do everything you can do to take your performance to a higher level and "get noticed."

Plyometrics for Athletes at All Levels is your guide to implementing this cutting-edge training method. Run faster, jump higher and be as quick as you want to be. Whether you're a recreational soccer player or a masters-level weekend warrior, let plyometrics be your tool for success.

In simplest terms, plyometrics are exercises that involve a jumping, leaping or hopping movement. To understand how plyometrics works, let's take a close look at how your body operates. Muscles and tendons are similar to rubber bands. When you stretch a rubber band, you store elastic energy so that when you release one end of the rubber band, it suddenly and rapidly contracts back to its normal shorter length. But can elastic energy actually produce greater force than an active muscular contraction?

Take your hand and place it flat on a table or desk. Keeping your hand flat and still, raise only your middle finger

up off the table and purpose-fully "slam" it down onto the table. Do it a couple of times, gauging the force with which you are "tapping" the table with your finger. Then, keeping the rest of your hand flat on the table, use your opposite hand to quickly pull the same middle finger up off the table and allow it to snap back down onto the table. Do it a couple of times, assessing the force of the finger slapping down onto the table. You can clearly see that the stretching back of the finger results in greater force generation than simply lifting and actively contracting the finger.

Plyometric activities enable a muscle to reach maximal

force in the shortest amount of time. They promote quick, powerful movements using a "pre-stretch," or counter movement, involving something known as *stretch-shortening cycle*, which is discussed below. By using a combination of stored elastic energy in the muscles and tendons as well as the stretch reflex, plyometric exercises increase the power of subsequent movements.

Natural Reflexes

Your nervous and muscular systems work together to generate additional force. We have all experienced going to the doctor for a physical and having our "reflexes" checked. The doctor typically uses a rubber mallet to tap the patellar ligament in the middle of our knee and, in response, our foot naturally "kicks" forward. This is known as the myotatic, or stretch, reflex. The tapping of the ligament actually stretches the patello-femoral tendon and the quadriceps muscle.

The quadriceps, like other skeletal muscles, are made up of special muscle fibers— extrafusal and intrafusal muscle fibers. The intrafusal fibers have a very specialized purpose. These unique fibers contain what are known as muscle spindles, which have spiral-shaped nerve endings that sense the degree of stretch of that muscle fiber, as well as the rate of stretch, or how fast that fiber is stretching. This is crucial because the muscle spindles respond to the stretching, or lengthening, of the muscle by signaling to your spinal cord that the muscle is being stretched. In milliseconds, a signal returns to the muscle, telling the extrafusal fibers to autonomously contract, preventing or decelerating further stretching. Consider these mechanisms a "safety valve," sensing excessive or perhaps dangerous stretching of the muscle and almost instantaneously preventing further stretching from occurring.

So now we see that there is force resulting from elastic energy, as well as an "unconscious" contraction in a muscle as a result from stretching that muscle. What happens if we also consciously contract the muscle upon being stretched? Let's go back to our example of your middle finger. Place the same hand back down flat on the table. Try quickly pulling the same middle finger up off the table—just as you stretch the finger back, purposefully contract the flexors of the finger to slam it down onto the table. This is what happens during a plyometric activity. It is the perfect preparation and coordination of all these tools that will result in maximal force application.

Stretch-shortening Cycle

Let's now go back to the stretch-shortening cycle. The stretch-shortening cycle is simply the process that a muscle goes through as it stretches and then contracts during these types of movement. There are different phases of the stretch-shortening cycle. The first phase is the *eccentric phase*, when the muscle stretches or lengthens, thus storing elastic energy and stimulating the muscle spindles. The second phase is called the *amortization phase*; during this phase, signals are sent to the spinal cord and then via motor neurons back

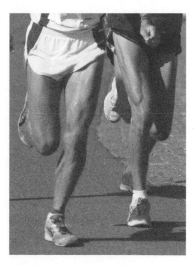

towards the extrafusal fibers. The third phase is the *concentric phase*, when the muscle actually responds to the previous two phases. It is during the concentric phase that the energy stored in the muscle "retracts," increasing the force production. This phenomenon is coupled with the reflexive muscle action resulting from the stretch reflex. When you add your conscious explosive contraction, the end result is significantly greater force application than would have resulted from simply contracting the muscle.

Consider a wildlife program you've seen that showed a herd of zebras grazing in the grasslands of Africa. When a lion came shooting out of the tall grass, hoping to catch its next meal, the initial reaction of the zebras was to bend down quickly and only slightly before exploding away from the lion and running for their lives. This is a demonstration of the stretch-shortening cycle. The quick stretch as the zebras lowered their center of gravity (eccentrically loading their muscles) set them up to dash away from the lion (concentric phase).

An important point to keep in mind is that if the muscle is stretched and held, the elastic energy is lost and dissipates as

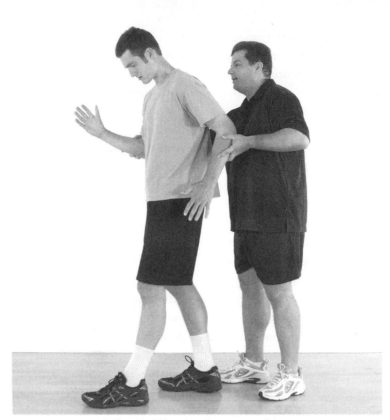

Author Neal Pire gives Sam some pointers.

heat. Thus any such stretch needs to be reversed suddenly and quickly in order to take advantage of this phenomenon. This can be demonstrated by squatting down before jumping, which allows the quadriceps to be stretched eccentrically so that the following concentric contraction will be stronger. If you squat down and hold the position for a second or two, and then jump, you simply can't produce the same explosive results. Research has shown that the faster the muscle is stretched eccentrically, the greater the force will be on

the following concentric contraction. The amount of tension created by stretching the muscle is dependent on the degree and the speed of the pre-stretch of that muscle.

Different Types of Plyometrics

Before we get into the "how-to," let's look at the wide array of plyometric exercises that you have at your fingertips.

Single-Effort vs. Multiple Jumps

You can perform plyometrics as single-effort or multiple jumps. *Single-effort jumps* are jumps that you perform once, reset and repeat for your desired number of repetitions. *Multiple jumps* are done in rapid succession for your desired number of repetitions. Either of these types of jumps may be performed over barriers, such as cones or hurdles, to help accelerate overall power development and enhances the lower body's ability to decelerate and change direction explosively. They can be performed in any chosen direction, forward and backward, side to side, on a diagonal, or in multiple pre-planned or random directions to make the exercises more difficult and enhance different movement-pattern develop-ment. You can perform them for a set number of repetitions, or you can do as many as you can for a set period of time.

Skill Combinations

Skill combinations are an ideal way to make your drills even more sport-specific. They inte-grate an agility skill with a sport-specific movement. You do these by combining any plyometric exercise with other movement skills to increase difficulty, add variety and incorporate more sport-specific movements. Some examples: perform a counter-movement jump and immediately upon landing sprint five yards; set up a box under a basketball rim, per-form a depth jump off the box and jump up towards the rim upon landing; perform a standing broad jump then immediately cut to the left and sprint for five yards upon landing. You can even com-bine lower- and upper-body plyometric exercises. One combination might be to execute a 90-degree jump, catch a medicine ball upon landing and immediately per-form a plyometric chest pass. Your options are endless.

Jumps in Place

With these, you land in the same place that you start from. These jumps should be maxi-mum effort and, like all exercises, should emphasize correct jumping technique and speed of movement. They're great for teaching you optimal jumping and landing technique, as well as explosive movement.

Standing Jumps

These refer to single-effort or multiple jumps that result in moving in any one direction. They require explosive move-ment and are ideal for developing lower-body power. They should be done with maximum effort and should emphasize correct technique and speed of movement.

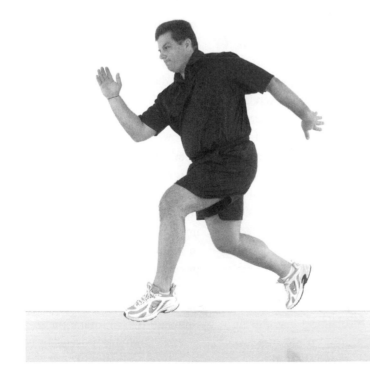

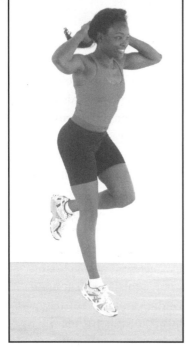

benefits of plyometrics

Now that you know what plyometric exercise is and basically how it works at the muscular level, what can it do for you? Before we answer the question, let's look at the history of plyometrics. Plyometrics is not a new fad or the latest training craze. It has a history, albeit brief, of demonstrated success in the international arena of world-class athletes.

In the early 1960s, Soviet researchers who were assigned the task of improving their athletes' performance began promoting training programs that involved using the stretch reflex. They referred to this type of training as "plyometric," which comes from two Greek words meaning "more" and "to measure." They used this term to describe the greater tension that could be developed in muscles when a quick stretching phase is followed by a fast contraction.

In 1966, Soviet jumping coach Yuri Verkhoshansky, wrote about the need to find a new way of improving athletic performance. Traditional training methods that combined resistance training with a high volume of jumping exercises were becoming less effective. Verkhoshansky observed that those jumpers that spent the least amount of ground contact time (amortization phase) showed the greatest jumping performance. He concluded that optimal jumping performance needed muscles to be strong eccentrically so that they could withstand the high mechanical load during amortization. If muscles were strong eccentrically, they

would be able to quickly switch from overcoming the eccentric loading to immediately contracting concentrically to accelerate the body in the required direction. This would allow the athlete to take advantage of the tension in the muscle that was created during the eccentric stretch. He reasoned that improvements could be made in jumping performance by increasing the amount of tension the athlete could generate during the eccentric contraction, and by improving the reactive ability of muscles in switching from eccentric to concentric work. This was done by performing "depth jumps," or jumping down from an elevated surface (off a box, for instance) and immediately jumping upward upon landing. Depth jumps became the tool of choice to accomplish this, evolving into a mainstay in Soviet training circles.

In the mid-1970s, track-and-field coach Fred Wilt was the first to write about plyometrics in the United States. He introduced plyometrics as a training technique used by European coaches to bridge the gap between strength and speed. This led to the widespread use of plyometrics in track and field in the United States. It also led to a heated debate regarding the efficacy and safety of plyometrics for improving athletic performance.

Plyometrics has since become the sports coach's tool to enhance athletes' running speed, jumping ability and overall agility. Athleticism, in general, can be dramatically improved with the effective use of plyometrics.

Sport Specificity

Most sports require a blend of athletic abilities. Among these are *straight-ahead speed* (a combination of acceleration and maximum velocity), *sport-speed* (the ability to change direction quickly and explosively) and *power* (typically expressed as jumping power, or a single explosive sport-specific skill like throwing a javelin in track and field, or suplexing your opponent onto the mat in wrestling). Upper-body athleticism falls into a similar continuum. Some sports such as football and basketball require *push-pull power*, while others require more *rotational power*, like baseball and golf. The chart

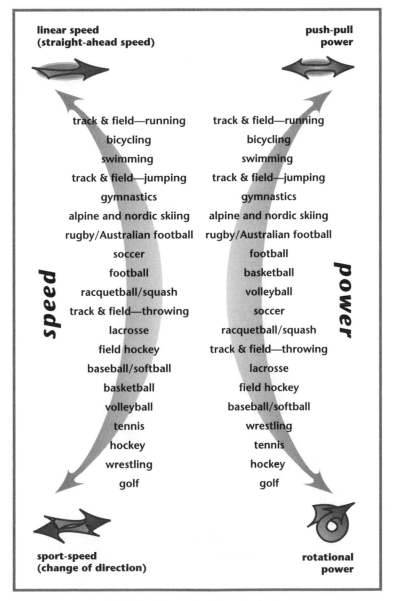

Speed and Power Continuum in Sports

on page 13 describes the speed and power continuum in sports. Take a look to see where your sport falls within the range of possibilities.

Some sports emphasize one ability over another. For example, training for a sprinter or long jumper in track and field should emphasize more acceleration and power development than agility, while conditioning for soccer should focus significantly more on agility. By performing the correct balance of plyometric exercises, you can enhance the abilities for your sport.

Maximizing Results

Research focusing specifically on the effectiveness of plyometric exercises done by themselves versus using plyometrics simultaneously with a resistance program has concluded that the best training results come when resistance training is combined with plyometric work. Combining plyometrics with strength training is the most effective method to maximize power development because it allows more physiological components of explosive power to be developed.

Some coaches believe that a typical resistance-training session should include plyometric work such as squat jumps and medicine ball drills in between resistance-training exercises. The objective is to achieve high-velocity movements mixed in with the resistance-training work. Other coaches believe that resistance training and plyometrics should not be combined during the same session. The bottom line is that most experts agree that resistance training and plyometrics should be combined in some form, whether it is in the same session or on alternate days. You should decide which works best for you.

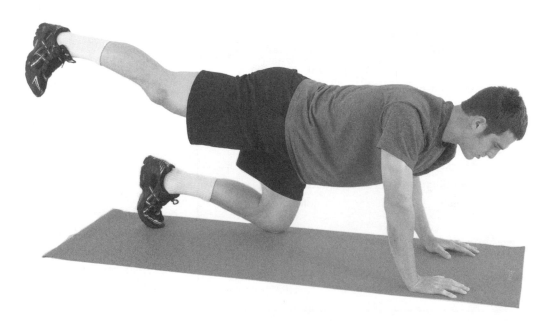

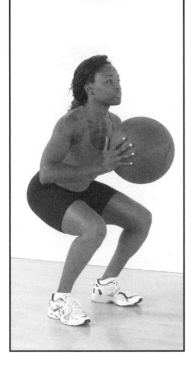

safety issues

For all of the positive press that plyometrics has received, there has been considerable criticism as well. Exercises such as depth jumping have been criticized as putting too much strain on the joints of the lower body and placing the athlete at risk of leg injuries. Famed Dallas Cowboy team orthopedist, Dr. Pat Evan, claimed that he saw more medical problems caused from depth jumping than from any other drill.

Other training professionals have criticized plyometrics as dangerous, with several well-known athletes blaming high-intensity plyometrics as having a negative impact on their careers. John Brenner, for example, a bronze medalist shot putter in the 1987 World Games, detached his quadriceps muscle performing a depth jump.

But is plyometrics itself the danger, or improper use of this training tool? Peter Tegen, head track coach at the University of Wisconsin, maintains that the numerous injuries sustained by athletes in the West from plyometric training is a result of too much too soon. He points out that in the Eastern block countries, athletes progressed through all of their training in very distinct stages, from small jumping exercises to depth jumps, and these activities were introduced after the athlete had developed a significant base of requisite strength and movement skills. U.S. Air Force Academy strength and conditioning coach Kim Gross reportedly suggested that many of the injuries from plyometrics occur because athletes and coaches do not realize how intense the exercises are.

It is important to closely monitor the length and frequency of plyometric workouts. There have been no epidemiological studies to suggest that the injury rates associated with using plyometrics is significant. In fact, plyometrics can be used to prevent pre-season soreness, and has been found to help reduce the incidence of anterior cruciate ligament (ACL) injuries in female athletes.

The general consensus among coaches is that plyometric training can be used

NSCA POSITION STATEMENT

It is the position of the National Strength and Conditioning Association that:

1. The stretch-shortening cycle, characterized by a rapid deceleration of a mass followed almost immediately by rapid acceleration of the mass in the opposite direction, is essential in the performance of most competitive sports, particularly those involving running, jumping and rapid changes in direction.

2. A plyometric exercise program which trains the muscles, connective tissue and nervous system to effectively carry out the stretch-shortening cycle can improve performance in most competitive sports.

3. A plyometric training program for athletes should include sport-specific exercises.

4. Carefully applied plyometric exercise programs are no more harmful than other forms of sports training and competition, and may be necessary for safe adaptation to the rigors of explosive sports.

5. Only athletes who have already achieved high levels of strength through standard resistance training should engage in plyometric drills.

6. Depth jumps should only be used by a small percentage of athletes engaged in plyometric training. As a rule, athletes weighing over 220 lbs. should not depth jump from platforms higher than 18 inches.

7. Plyometric drills involving a particular muscle/joint complex should not be performed on consecutive days.

8. Plyometric drills should not be performed when an athlete is fatigued. Time for complete recovery should be allowed between plyometric exercise sets.

9. Footwear and landing surfaces used in plyometric drills must have good shock-absorbing qualities.

10. A thorough set of warm-up exercises should be performed before beginning a plyometric training session. Less demanding drills should be mastered prior to attempting more complex and intense drills.

Position Statement: Explosive/Plyometric Exercises. National Strength & Conditioning Association Journal: Vol. 15, No. 3, pp. 16, 1993.

with adolescent athletes as long as these exercises are performed with low volume and intensity. Jumps should be off of both feet with no added stimulus of weights or boxes. Conditioning coach Vern Gambetta has suggested that plyometric training should progress from simple to complex as the athlete matures. This means going from bouncing movements, standing jumps to short jumps, and then finally progressing to depth jumps. He stresses that depth jumping should only be used if technique is sound and adequate strength levels have been achieved. Rules of thumb exist, suggesting that an athlete needs to be able to back squat 1.5 to 2.5 times their body weight before participating in advanced plyometric exercises. The table on this page outlines the National Strength and Conditioning Association's (NSCA) position statement on plyometrics, which provides a simple list of guidelines.

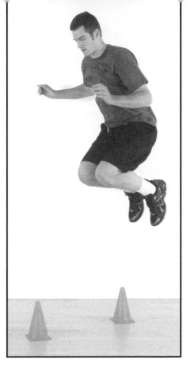

before you begin

This section will provide some basic rules of thumb to help you get the most out of your plyometrics workouts, while minimizing any potential risks of injury. You will also find a brief description of the "tools of the trade"— equipment commonly used in plyometric exercise.

Prerequisites

The National Strength and Conditioning Association (NSCA) guidelines indicate that, for lower body plyometrics, you should be able to perform one perfect parallel squat (1 repetition maximum, or 1RM) with at least one and a half times your body weight. Other experts recommend a 1RM parallel squat with at least 75 percent of your body weight, or a timed five-repetition set of the parallel squat at 60 percent of your body weight within five seconds. For upper body plyometrics, they recommend five "clap" push-ups. Before we continue analyzing these guidelines, I'd like to share some food for thought with you.

Since you now understand what plyometrics are, would you not classify a simple skip as a plyometric exercise? How about running? The fact is that almost every athletic activity has plyometric movements inherent in the activity. Sprinting can be described as a series of plyometric leaps, with an eccentric phase, a short amortization phase and a concentric response driving your center of gravity forward, quickly and explosively. It's not the plyometric nature of the movements that impose a prerequisite. Rather, it's the intensity of each movement that indicates whether or not

you should indulge in a particular plyometric exercise.

To solve the "are you ready?" dilemma, I recommend that you look at two things as your litmus tests for clearance to perform plyometric exercises:

1) You should be at least three months into a progressive resistance-training program. *There is no substitute for strength!* Ultimately, the stronger you are, the more force you can apply into the ground, which will inevitably produce more powerful movement. What plyometric drills do is bring the nervous system "up to speed" so you get the most out of whatever strength you do have. Logically speak-

ing, you should be able to perform a perfect parallel back squat with your body weight loaded on the bar prior to considering a comprehensive plyometrics program, but not being able to do so *should not* preclude you from performing basic plyometric drills. Remember that if you participate in sports like basketball, soccer or softball, you are already performing explosive movements that require you to move quickly and forcefully, and decelerate suddenly.

2) The second "test" is the most important. Can you perform the given plyometric exercise *perfectly*? Form is always important when you exercise, but when you move quickly and explosively, the stress on your joints and body overall is significant. If you can't maintain proper alignment while landing a jump (such that your hips, knees and ankles are aligned), and, for example, your knees "cave in" as you absorb the impact of landing the jump, you should not be performing that particular exercise.

Equipment

It's possible to follow an effective, progressive plyometrics program using nothing but your body weight and the space you have available. However, there are some tools that will help you add variety to your program. Most of the equipment listed below can be found at the bigger sporting-goods retailers or at various online fitness-equipment retailers accessible via a simple online search.

Hurdles and Cones

Cones provide you with a target, a mark or a barrier with which to work with. *Saucer cones* are very close to the ground and are ideal for drills that require you to touch the cones with your hands. This forces you to keep your center of gravity very low to the ground, which is ideal for many sports, such as basketball. You can use *standard cones* ranging in height from 6 inches to 18 inches as barriers to move around or jump over. You can also use *hurdle*

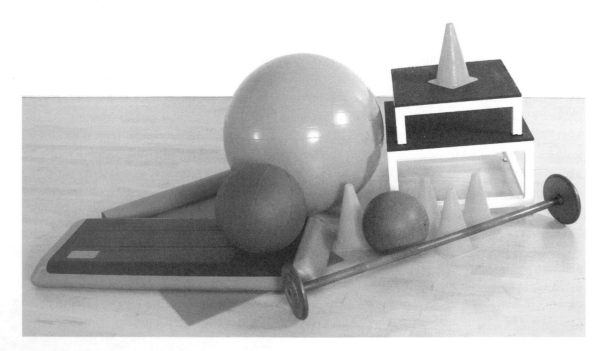

cones that come with poles and clips to provide barriers to move over, under and around.

Traditional track-and-field **hurdles** are useful barriers for explosive hopping drills, but tend to present some inherent risk because of their rigid construction. Some newer versions designed specifically for plyometric drills and conditioning are adjustable from 6 to 42 inches, and offer a variety of uses from hurdle walks to plyometric bounding, jumping and hopping. In addition to collapsibility (a good safety feature), they are portable, easily folding up for storage. In this book, any exercise using a cone can also be done with a hurdle. Jumping over hurdles or cones develops overall power and enhances the lower body's ability to decelerate and change direction explosively.

Plyo Boxes

Plyo boxes typically range from 6 to 30 inches in height. They have a sturdy design and are stable enough to withstand you jumping up onto them. The landing surface or top of the box has a surface area of 18 by 24 inches and is made of a non-slip material. If you do not have a plyo box, you can substitute with an aerobics step or bench. Keep in mind, though, that plyo boxes are

designed specifically for these types of activities: they are stable and provide a perfect landing surface for jumps. Benches do not, and a step is nowhere nearly as stable as a plyo box.

Rings and Dots

Rings and **dots** simply serve as a "target" landing area for your foot or feet. You may draw these landing areas on the floor with chalk, or use masking tape to create targets in which to land each hop.

Medicine Balls

Medicine balls offer tremendous versatility for upper-body plyometric training. Not only can you use balls of a variety of weights and diameters, you can also use specially designed balls with single or double handles, balls that bounce when thrown against a hard surface, or balls that don't bounce at all.

Stability Balls

Stability balls have been used for years in physical rehabilitation. They're designed as a soft, supportive surface that will naturally challenge your balance and "wake up" your nervous system. They typically come in three or four sizes. Most people do well with a 55cm ball, but for taller ath-

letes, a 65cm might be best. To figure out what is ideal for you, your knees should be at a 90-degree angle when sitting upright on a fully inflated ball.

BOSU

The **BOSU** ("Bottom Side Up") is a hot item in sports and fitness conditioning these days. It looks like a stability ball cut in half. It'll challenge your balance without ever rolling out from under you as stability balls might. For optimal stimulus and safety, always be sure that stability balls and BOSUs are adequately inflated to manufacturer's recommendations.

Barbells

It should be safe to assume that you are already following a comprehensive resistance-training program, but so as not to leave any stone unturned, let's briefly talk about your **barbells**. There's a supplemental resistance-training exercise added to each plyometrics workout. Because of the nature of these explosive lifts, it is ideal to use an Olympic-style barbell for these exercises. The ends of these bars freely rotate around the bar, making it easy for you to perform the recommended lifts. This will maximize your performance during these lifts without undue stress on your wrists.

Ab Dolly

The **Ab Dolly** is designed as a functional abdominal training tool, but it also makes for a clever add-on to your plyometrics toolbox. It allows you to stabilize your legs while your arms perform, or otherwise. You'll surely find many uses for this simple yet innovative piece of exercise equipment.

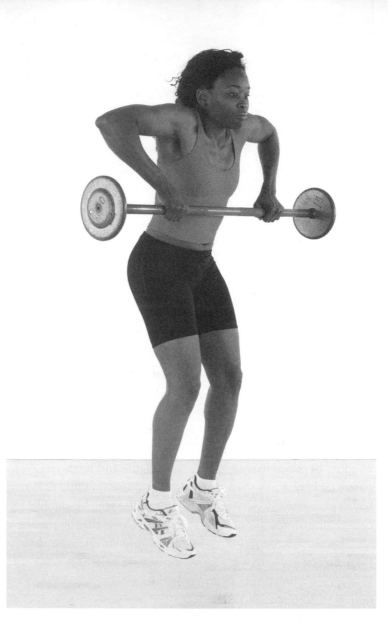

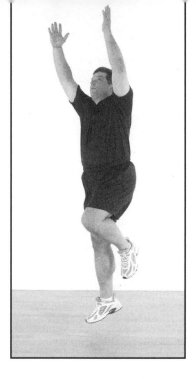

basic training principles

Like any other fitness training modality, there are some basic principles that you should consider when incorporating plyometrics into your conditioning program.

Intensity typically refers to the amount of stress placed on the involved muscles, connective tissue and joints, and is primarily dictated by the drills performed. Active dynamic warm-up exercises like Forward Skips and Carioca are lower-intensity movements, while Depth Jumps are higher-intensity exercises.

Frequency is the number of plyometric sessions per week, and typically ranges from one to three, depending on the athlete's level of conditioning, the sport and the in/off-season status of the athlete. The most important issue is *recovery*— there should be a period of 48 to 72 hours between plyometric training sessions. *Acute recovery* is also important:

It is crucial that you allow enough rest between repetitions and sets so as not to compromise the optimal form and performance of each exercise, thus risking injury and minimizing the effectiveness of the exercise.

Volume is typically measured by the total number of repetitions and sets during a given plyometric session. The unit of measurement is the actual number of foot contacts (hops) or distance covered during a given exercise (e.g., bounding). For upper-body plyometrics, the total number of throws per workout is measured. Here are some basic volume recommendations based specifically on your level of experience:

Beginner: 80–100 contacts
Intermediate: 100–120 contacts
Advanced: 120–140 contacts

When trying to map out your training plan, keep in mind that, as with any training program, you need to follow the basic principles of progressive overload. Intensity and volume are interactive. As your intensity goes up, you might want to decrease your volume, and vice versa. In time you will find the optimal combination of these program-design variables to get the most out of your plyometrics conditioning program.

The Big Picture

The beauty of *Plyometrics for Athletes at All Levels* is that it provides you with a simple approach to getting started. In Part 2 you'll find three levels of programs (beginner, intermediate, advanced) tailored to specific sports.

Always start with the Dynamic Warm-Up & Muscle-Activation Series on pages 28–29 before moving on to your specific program. The muscle-activation exercises enhance mobilization of muscles such as the psoas and piriformis, which are important in athleticism. Some of these muscles act as stabilizers, preventing unwanted movement. Others are primary movers, acting as agonists, or muscles that move the limb as you desire through one portion of a movement, and then immediately serving as an antagonist, or a muscle that opposes your desired movement, thus requiring it to relax so as not to interfere with your desired movement.

Being able to complete this progression of plyometric exercises without feeling excessively fatigued will tell you what kind of shape you are in. For many, completing just the first two portions of the progression is a challenge. Don't be fooled into thinking you can just move on to more intense progressions if you are spent just after the warm-up and muscle-activation series.

Be smart and safe to get faster, jump higher and EXPLODE!

Proper Form

Precise form of all plyometric exercises is crucial to preventing injury and getting the most out of your exercises. For one thing, *never* lock your knees. If your form starts to deteriorate in a training session, then the exercise should be stopped. For example, listen for "loud landings," which signify that you're not absorbing the impact of your landings. Other signs of deteriorating form are slow, sluggish movement instead of quick, crisp movements, and undesired mechanics like knees buckling in upon landing jumps.

It's important that ground contact time (amortization phase) be as short as possible. If you're spending too much time on the ground, move on to the next exercise. Remember, quality over quantity.

Athletic Ready Position

As children, we've all heard "Stand up straight," "Don't slouch" and/or "Keep your chin up." The fact is that there's an ideal posture for every activity, whether you're sitting at a desk typing, standing at attention hour-on-end guarding Buckingham Palace, or taking your opponent to the hole on the basketball court.

Ideal posture when standing is when the body achieves optimal balance. It requires very little muscular activity to maintain. Your spine is in its natural "neutral" state, your knees almost "locked," and your head balanced on top of your shoulders. You can stand in this highly efficient position for a very long time without fatiguing. Similarly, when performing in sports, there's an ideal body position that maximizes your ability to perform—the athletic ready position.

To assume the athletic ready position, you stand on the balls of your feet with

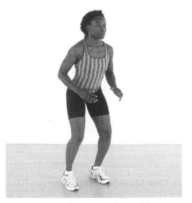

Correct athletic ready position

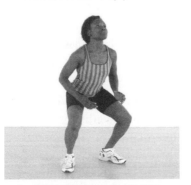

Incorrect athletic ready position: too much arch in back and neck

your feet a little wider than shoulder-width apart, keeping your back straight. You're slightly flexed at the ankles, knees and hips. This prepares you to eccentrically load your hips and legs so you can burst into a sprint or jump. Your hands are in front of your body with your elbows relaxed and flexed. Your head is up, eyes forward. You are now ready to EXPLODE!

Learning to automatically assume the athletic ready position at all times while playing your sport will enhance your first-step quickness, your ability to change direction, and your ability to jump skyward.

Quadruped

When in quadruped position, or on your hands and knees, make sure your hands are directly under your shoulders and your knees are directly under your hips. This creates a stable foundation.

Rhythmic breathing

Breathe naturally and rhythmically while performing your

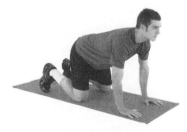

Quadruped position

plyometrics workout progressions. Be conscious of your breathing patterns. Don't hold your breath. Allow your body to naturally gravitate to the breathing pattern it chooses throughout all the exercises.

Progression

You should progress gradually from basic plyometric exercises to more intense drills. The intensity and volume of your plyometric work should always be *right for you*. If you have not built the requisite foundation of strength, you should wait before performing more intense drills.

Stretching

Stretching is an invaluable tool in sports conditioning. The benefits of regular, progressive stretching are significant. That said, it is strongly recommended that all stretching be left to the end of your workout. Static stretching prior to sports activities has been shown to be detrimental to performance. To get the most out of your plyometrics exercises and your flexibility training, follow this order: warm-up, muscle activation, plyometrics progressions, static stretching/cool-down.

Common Mistakes

All too often our minds and hearts are so full of the desire

to excel that we cross the line or do something foolish that actually slows our progress. Don't think that more is always better. "No pain, no gain" is not appropriate in this case.

To avoid injury, you are always best off performing the exercises as recommended in your sport-specific Rx, but only *after* you've finished the Dynamic Warm-Up & Muscle-Activation Series. Even if you are already warmed up from prior exercise, the warm-up and muscle-activation series prepares your muscles, joints and nervous system for your plyometrics progression. Your ability to perform will be heightened by completing this progression, and this will ensure that you will get the most out of your plyometrics workout.

Perform only the total number of contacts that are recommended in each Rx. Don't perform additional sets or exercises if you happen to feel "fresh" during a given workout. Precise performance of all movements is paramount so make sure that you have adequately recovered between exercises or sets. Remember that you don't improve during your workouts—you improve in between workouts during your rest days, so be sure to get ample rest.

part two:

the

programs

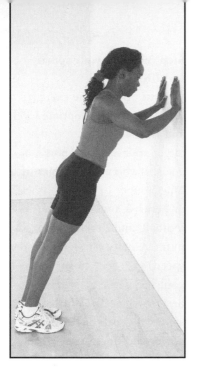

your plyometrics Rx

No matter what your level of conditioning or experience, or sport-specific goals, you will get the results you are looking for if you follow the right training program for you. The sample programs in this section target an array of athletes at different levels of conditioning. Use these as your guide to implementing this cutting-edge training technique.

Specialize It

Designing the right program is simple, much like putting pieces of a puzzle together. The recommended workouts in *Plyometrics for Athletes at All Levels* take a lot of the guesswork out of program design for your particular sport, making it easy to weave plyometrics into your regular sports-conditioning regimen. Each workout addresses the inherent needs of your sport, and is split up into three four-week phases, providing the right stimuli to take you to a higher performance level.

Plyometric exercises should be specific to your sport. For instance, upper-body plyometrics drills would be more relevant for a football player than for a figure skater. Similarly, speed skaters and athletes who require quick changes of direction would benefit from plyometric exercises that challenge lateral acceleration. Be sure to choose the workout that best suits your sport, and be sure to perform these and all of your exercises with the utmost quality in mind. This is the only way to achieve

optimal results from your training.

Begin each workout with the Dynamic Warm-Up & Muscle-Activation Series on pages 28–29 to help prepare your joints, muscles and nervous system for the challenges presented by plyometrics. Then you're ready to roll on to the sport-specific drills.

Step 1: Select the program based on your primary sport (the sport you are currently training for).

If you are a two-sport athlete, however, and you play

baseball in the spring/summer and basketball in the fall/winter, decide which sport you will predominantly be playing 12 weeks from the start of your plyometrics program. Then select that program.

Step 2: Select an exercise level appropriate to your abilities.

If you are new to plyometrics, or if you have been following a resistance-training program but have not performed plyometric exercises in the past three months, you should select the *Beginner Plyometrics Workout* (page 31), regardless of the sport you play. If you have been strength training and have had some experience performing plyo-

metric exercises in at least the past three months, you should select the *Intermediate* workout for your chosen sport. If you are a high-level athlete, or have been following an intensive strength-training program as well as performing plyometric exercises on a regular basis, you should select the *Advanced* workout. These are exercise selection guidelines and do not supersede the "Prerequisites" outlined on pages 17–18. As explained on page 22, you should perform the Dynamic Warm-Up & Muscle-Activation Series prior to every plyometrics session. *Do not just go straight into your plyometrics series without completing these sequences!*

Step 3: Select your sport-specific goal.

Next, look at the exercises listed at your appropriate level and then select those that target your specific sport goals. If you are a sprinter or long jumper in track and field, or perhaps a wide receiver in football, and developing maximum velocity (straight-ahead speed) is crucial to success in your sport, select exercises designated as *Speed*. If you are a volleyball or basketball player and developing jumping and leaping ability is important to your athletic success, select exercises designated as *Jump*. If you are a soccer or lacrosse player, or if sport-speed (the ability to cut and change direction quickly and explosively) is vital to you, then select exercises that are designated as *COD* (change of direction). This type of exercise is perfect for developing overall agility. Similarly, choose the exercises that target your upper-body goal: *Rotational Power* or *Push-Pull Power*.

Keep in mind that most sports require a combination of athletic abilities. Few sports (such as the 100-meter sprint) require unique attributes and not much of others, and some sports will require different combinations based on your position on the team. If you

SOME TERMS DEFINED

LEVEL I: Beginner   Ideal for the athlete who has been following a strength-training program but has not performed plyometrics in the past 3 months.

LEVEL II: Intermediate   Ideal for the athlete who has been strength training and has had some experience performing plyometric exercises for at least the past 3 months.

LEVEL III: Advanced   Ideal for the experienced athlete who has been strength training and has been performing plyometric exercises on a regular basis.

SPEED   Exercise that is ideal for developing "maximum velocity," or straight-ahead speed. Perfect for

sprinters, football wide receivers.

JUMPING   Exercise that is ideal for developing jumping and leaping ability. Perfect for volleyball and basketball players.

COD (Change of Direction)   Exercise that is optimal for developing "sport speed," that is, the ability to cut and change direction quickly and explosively. This type of exercise is perfect for developing overall agility.

PUSH-PULL POWER   Power that emphasizes explosive force directly forward, overhead or backward.

ROTATIONAL POWER   Power that emphasizes explosive force across the body, ideal for explosive trunk and hip rotation.

play football, for example, an offensive lineman will be required to change direction often but will occasionally need to sprint downfield. This athlete's plyometrics prescription might be a total of six exercises, including five COD exercises and one Speed exercise.

Step 4: Now do it.

Begin your workout with the Dynamic Warm-Up & Muscle-Activation Series on pages 28–29 before tackling your sport-specific program (remember that if you are new to plyometrics, you will be doing the Beginner Plyometrics Workout on page 31). Each exercise listed in your personal prescription has a number of sets and contacts, with a suggested recovery period. Keep in mind that if you rest the recommended 2 to 3 minutes between sets, and your form in subsequent sets

is not as "perfect" as your first set, you may need to lengthen your recovery period between sets of that exercise. It is preferable to add to your recovery time and perform your plyometric exercises precisely, as you should, than it is to keep to the recommended recoveries and watch your form deteriorate as you fatigue throughout the workout.

You can proceed through the sequence of exercises and then repeat the sequence when multiple sets are prescribed, or perform the multiple sets back-to-back, and then proceed to the next exercise.

You should do each level for four weeks before progressing to the next one. After completing a full cycle of your plyometrics program (progressing through Beginner, Intermediate, and Advanced), you may weave in and replace the pre-designed series with other similar exercises (see "Fine-Tuning It" below).

Fine-Tuning It

After completing your assigned plyometrics prescription at least once, you might decide that you want to change an exercise. You may substitute a recommended exercise for another. Just make sure that the particular exercise you choose is similar in level and emphasis. For example, if you

want to substitute an exercise for Slalom Hops, which is a Level I exercise with a focus on change of direction, you may select One-Legged Slalom Hops, an exercise that provides similar characteristics. An example for upper-body variations could be substituting Vertical Scoop Toss for the Back Toss. They are both Level II exercises that develop push-pull power.

Keep in mind that the suggested level for each exercise is relative and is only specific to your ability to perform the exercise. You might find it difficult to perform a Level I exercise that requires lateral stability, but have no problem with a Level III exercise that emphasizes linear velocity. The suggested levels are solely a general guide to help you devise a progression—that is, which exercises you should be able to do before you move up to the next level of exercises.

Citius, Altius, Fortius

You now have the tools you need to take your athletic performance to a new level. Follow the guidelines in *Plyometrics for Athletes at All Levels* and you will live the Olympic motto: *Citius, Altius, Fortius*—Latin for "Swifter, Higher, Stronger."

Work hard, good luck and EXPLODE!

warm-up & muscle-activation series

All athletes, regardless of fitness level, should start their workout with this series. The warm-up drills will help your body "learn" how to perform in these very specific movement patterns, which will help you achieve more efficient motor skills and further enhance your athleticism. The muscle-activation exercises are designed to enhance mobilization of the muscles that are important in athletics.

DYNAMIC WARM-UP & MUSCLE-ACTIVATION SERIES

	PAGE	EXERCISE	SETS	CONTACTS/ DISTANCE	RECOVERY (seconds)		
					Beg.	Int.	Adv.
all sports	74	forward skips	1	10 yds	10	5	None
	75	prisoner squats	1	10 cntcs	10	5	None
	76	forward hurdler skips	1	10 yds	10	5	None
	77	alternating side squats	1	10 cntcs	10	5	None
	78	backward hurdler skips	1	10 yds	10	5	None
	79	alternating rear lunges	1	10 cntcs	10	5	None
	80	lateral shuffle	1	10 yds	10	5	None
	81	alternating lateral lunges	1	10 cntcs	10	5	None
	82	carioca	1	10 yds	10	5	None

DYNAMIC WARM-UP & MUSCLE-ACTIVATION SERIES

	PAGE	EXERCISE	SETS	CONTACTS/ DISTANCE	RECOVERY (seconds)		
					Beg.	Int.	Adv.
	83	gate swings	1	10 cntcs	10	5	None
	84	backward cycle run	1	10 yds	10	5	None
	85	supine leg raises	1	10 cntcs	5	3	None
	86	lateral leg raises	1	10 cntcs	5	3	None
	87	inside leg raises	1	10 cntcs	5	3	None
	88	hydrants	1	10 cntcs	5	3	None
	89	forward circles on all fours	1	10 cntcs	5	3	None
	90	backward circles on all fours	1	10 cntcs	5	3	None
	91	kneeling kickbacks	1	10 cntcs	5	3	None
	92	seated hip thrusts	1	10 cntcs	5	3	None
	93	one-legged hip thrusts	1	10 cntcs		3	None

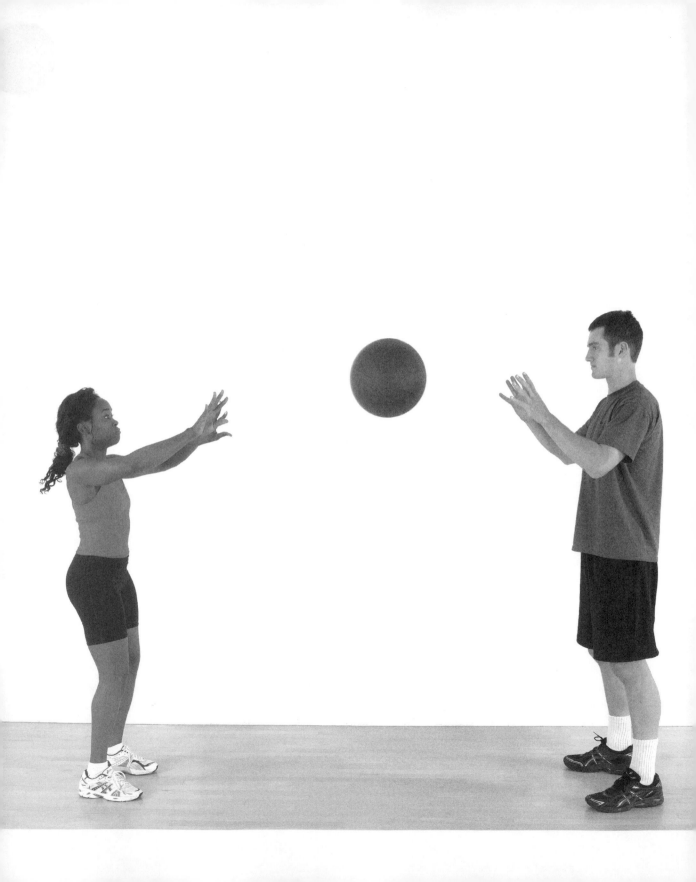

beginner plyometrics workout

Before you start this Level 1 workout, be sure to complete the Dynamic Warm-Up & Muscle-Activation Series on pages 28–29.

This workout is designed for athletes of any sport who are either new to plyometrics or who have been following a strength-training program but have not performed plyomet-

rics in the past three months. When doing this workout, you may choose to do Push-Ups on page 120 instead of Push-Ups (off the Wall) as noted below.

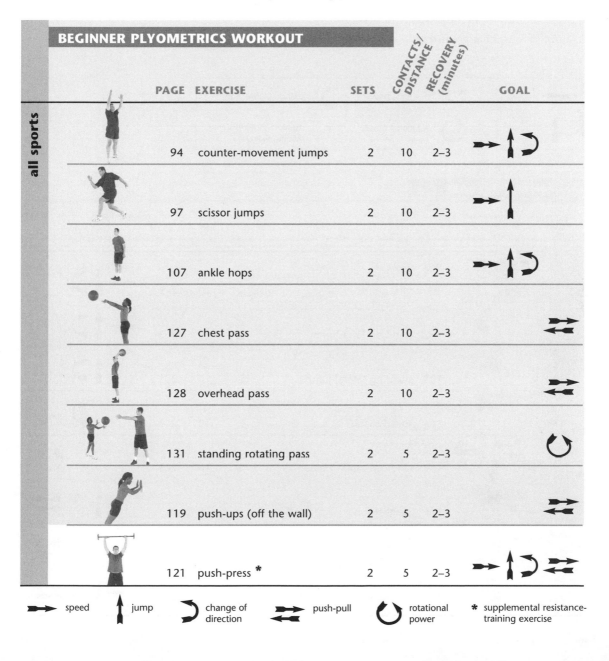

		PAGE	EXERCISE	SETS	CONTACTS/ DISTANCE	RECOVERY (minutes)	GOAL
all sports		94	counter-movement jumps	2	10	2–3	
		97	scissor jumps	2	10	2–3	
		107	ankle hops	2	10	2–3	
		127	chest pass	2	10	2–3	
		128	overhead pass	2	10	2–3	
		131	standing rotating pass	2	5	2–3	
		119	push-ups (off the wall)	2	5	2–3	
		121	push-press *	2	5	2–3	

BEGINNER PLYOMETRICS WORKOUT

speed   jump   change of direction   push-pull   rotational power   * supplemental resistance-training exercise

baseball/softball

Baseball and softball place a huge emphasis on first-step quickness and acceleration. Trunk and hip rotation play a big part in swinging the bat as well as throwing, so rotational power should be the upper-body training focus; change-of-direction training can help develop powerful hips. Before you jump into this program, start your plyometrics workout with the Dynamic Warm-Up & Muscle-Activation Series on pages 28–29.

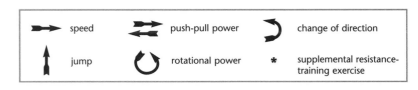

	speed		push-pull power		change of direction
	jump		rotational power	*	supplemental resistance-training exercise

INTERMEDIATE

	PAGE	EXERCISE	SETS	CONTACTS/ DISTANCE	RECOVERY (minutes)	GOAL
	99	tuck jumps	2	10	2–3	➤ ↑ ⤵
	102	standing broad jump	2	10	2–3	➤ ↑ ⤵
	103	standing lateral jump	2	10	2–3	↑ ⤵
	114	speed skaters	2	10	2–3	⤵
	132	lunging rotating pass	2	10	2–3	↻
	126	squat throws	2	10	2–3	↑ ⇄
	120	push-ups (level 2)	2	5	2–3	⇄
	122	high pulls *	2	5	2–3	➤ ↑ ⤵ ⇄

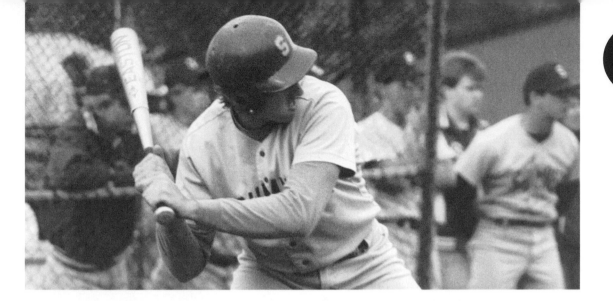

ADVANCED

	PAGE	EXERCISE	SETS	CONTACTS/ DISTANCE	RECOVERY (minutes)	GOAL
	115	alternating straddle hops	1	10	2–3	
	113	multiple hops over cones	2	10	2–3	
	103	standing lateral jump	2	10	2–3	
	114	speed skaters	2	10	2–3	
	116	box jumps	2	10	2–3	
	117	depth jumps	2	5	2–3	
	125	wood chops	2	10	2–3	
	136	rotational slams	2	10	2–3	
	137	vertical scoop toss	2	10	2–3	
	123	hanging cleans *	2	5	2–3	

basketball

Basketball emphasizes sport-speed, or change of direction, plus first-step quickness, acceleration and jumping ability. Upper-body requisites are primarily push-pull in nature, though explosive trunk rotation plays a big part in controlling the boards. Before you jump into this program, start your plyometrics workout with the Dynamic Warm-Up & Muscle-Activation Series on pages 28–29.

➤ speed	⬆ jump
⇄ push-pull power	↻ rotational power
⤴ change of direction	* supplemental resistance-training exercise

INTERMEDIATE

	PAGE	EXERCISE	SETS	CONTACTS/ DISTANCE	RECOVERY (minutes)	GOAL
	115	alternating straddle hops	2	10	2–3	➤ ⬆ ⤴
	108	bunny hops	2	10	2–3	⬆ ⤴
	106	90-degree jumps	2	10	2–3	⬆ ⤴
	114	speed skaters	2	10	2–3	⤴
	132	lunging rotating pass	2	10	2–3	↻
	126	squat throws	2	10	2–3	⬆ ⇄
	120	push-ups (level 2)	2	5	2–3	⇄
	122	high pulls *	2	5	2–3	➤ ⬆ ⤴ ⇄

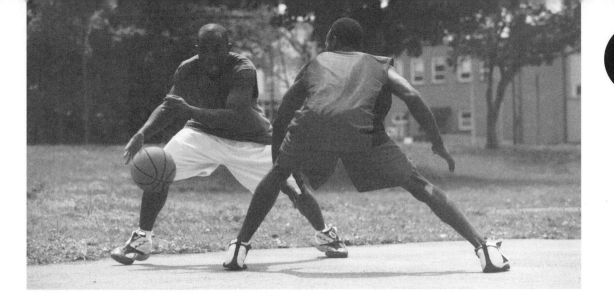

ADVANCED

	PAGE	EXERCISE	SETS	CONTACTS/ DISTANCE	RECOVERY (minutes)	GOAL
	118	box jump-ups	1	10	2–3	
	99	tuck jumps	2	10	2–3	
	113	multiple hops over cones	2	10	2–3	
	103	standing lateral jump	2	10	2–3	
	116	box jumps	2	10	2–3	
	117	depth jumps	2	5	2–3	
	125	wood chops	2	10	2–3	
	136	rotational slams	2	10	2–3	
	133	rotating pass on ball	2	10	2–3	
	123	hanging cleans *	2	5	2–3	

bicycling

Bicycling requires a tremendous amount of push-pull power, primarily in the lower body. A powerful core is necessary to utilize the lower body efficiently, so rotational power should be emphasized during upper-body training. Before you jump into this program, start your plyometrics workout with the Dynamic Warm-Up & Muscle-Activation Series on pages 28–29.

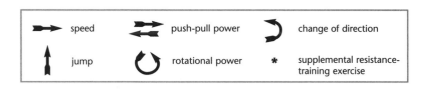

	speed		push-pull power		change of direction
	jump		rotational power	*	supplemental resistance-training exercise

INTERMEDIATE

	PAGE	EXERCISE	SETS	CONTACTS/DISTANCE	RECOVERY (minutes)	GOAL
	102	standing broad jump	2	10	2–3	
	97	scissor jumps	2	10	2–3	
	115	alternating straddle hops	2	10	2–3	
	100	counter-movement jumps, 1-leg	2	10	2–3	
	127	chest pass	2	10	2–3	
	126	squat throws	2	10	2–3	
	120	push-ups (level 2)	2	5	2–3	
	122	high pulls *	2	5	2–3	

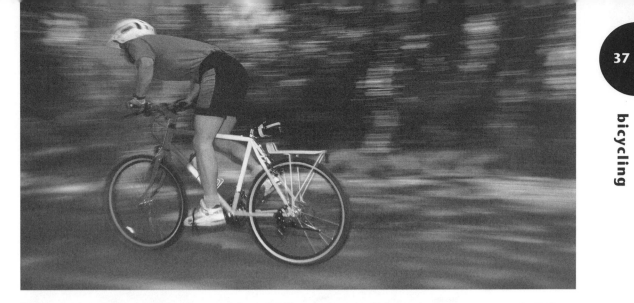

ADVANCED

	PAGE	EXERCISE	SETS	CONTACTS/DISTANCE	RECOVERY (minutes)	GOAL
	99	tuck jumps	1	10	2–3	
	118	box jump-ups	2	10	2–3	
	98	split jumps w/cycle	2	10	2–3	
	105	one-legged jumps	2	10	2–3	
	116	box jumps	2	10	2–3	
	117	depth jumps	2	5	2–3	
	125	wood chops	2	10	2–3	
	136	rotational slams	2	10	2–3	
	138	explosive start throws	2	10	2–3	
	123	hanging cleans *	2	5	2–3	

field hockey

Field hockey emphasizes sport-speed, or change of direction, as well as acceleration and first-step quickness. The upper-body requisite is primarily rotational power and explosiveness. Before you jump into this program, start your plyometrics workout with the Dynamic Warm-Up & Muscle-Activation Series on pages 28–29.

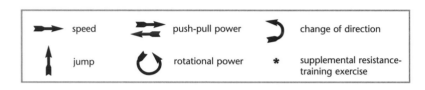

	speed		push-pull power		change of direction
	jump		rotational power	*	supplemental resistance-training exercise

INTERMEDIATE

	PAGE	EXERCISE	SETS	CONTACTS/DISTANCE	RECOVERY (minutes)	GOAL
	110	target hops	2	10	2–3	
	111	target hops (1 leg)	2	10	2–3	
	112	slalom hops (1 leg)	2	10	2–3	
	114	speed skaters	2	10	2–3	
	132	lunging rotating pass	2	10	2–3	
	139	back toss	2	10	2–3	
	120	push-ups (level 2)	2	5	2–3	
	122	high pulls *	2	5	2–3	

ADVANCED

	PAGE	EXERCISE	SETS	CONTACTS/ DISTANCE	RECOVERY (minutes)	GOAL
	99	tuck jumps	1	10	2–3	
	113	multiple hops over cones	2	10	2–3	
	103	standing lateral jump	2	10	2–3	
	105	one-legged jumps	2	10	2–3	
	116	box jumps	2	10	2–3	
	117	depth jumps	2	5	2–3	
	125	wood chops	2	10	2–3	
	136	rotational slams	2	10	2–3	
	138	explosive start throws	2	10	2–3	
	123	hanging cleans *	2	5	2–3	

football

Football generally emphasizes sport-speed, or change of direction, but explosiveness and first-step quickness are crucial to a player's success. Upper-body requisites have a slight emphasis on rotational power versus push-pull power, though both are important. Before you jump into this program, start your plyometrics workout with the Dynamic Warm-Up & Muscle-Activation Series on pages 28–29.

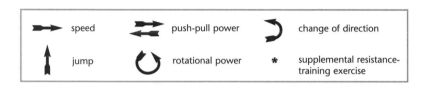

	speed		push-pull power		change of direction
	jump		rotational power	*	supplemental resistance-training exercise

INTERMEDIATE

	PAGE	EXERCISE	SETS	CONTACTS/ DISTANCE	RECOVERY (minutes)	GOAL
	102	standing broad jump	2	10	2–3	➤ ↑ ⤴
	97	scissor jumps	2	10	2–3	➤ ↑
	109	slalom hops	2	10	2–3	➤ ↑ ⤴
	114	speed skaters	2	10	2–3	⤴
	125	wood chops	2	10	2–3	↑ ⇄
	126	squat throws	2	10	2–3	↑ ⇄
	120	push-ups (level 2)	2	5	2–3	⇄
	122	high pulls *	2	5	2–3	➤ ↑ ⤴ ⇄

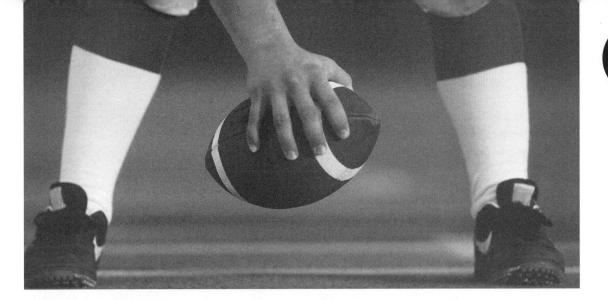

ADVANCED

	PAGE	EXERCISE	SETS	CONTACTS/ DISTANCE	RECOVERY (minutes)	GOAL
	99	tuck jumps	1	10	2–3	
	113	multiple hops over cones	2	10	2–3	
	103	standing lateral jump	2	10	2–3	
	105	one-legged jumps	2	10	2–3	
	116	box jumps	2	10	2–3	
	117	depth jumps	2	5	2–3	
	137	vertical scoop toss	2	10	2–3	
	136	rotational slams	2	10	2–3	
	138	explosive start throws	2	10	2–3	
	123	hanging cleans *	2	5	2–3	

golf

Golf places a huge emphasis on single-repetition explosiveness. Trunk and hip rotation play a significant role in golf, so rotational power should be the upper-body training focus, while change-of-direction training can help develop powerful hips. Before you jump into this program, start your plyometrics workout with the Dynamic Warm-Up & Muscle-Activation Series on pages 28–29.

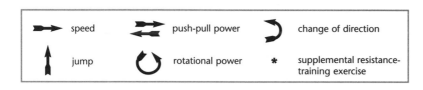

		speed			push-pull power			change of direction
		jump			rotational power	*		supplemental resistance-training exercise

INTERMEDIATE

	PAGE	EXERCISE	SETS	CONTACTS/DISTANCE	RECOVERY (minutes)	GOAL
	104	standing diagonal jump	2	10	2–3	↑ ⤴
	97	scissor jumps	2	10	2–3	→ ↑
	106	90-degree jumps	2	10	2–3	↑ ⤴
	114	speed skaters	2	10	2–3	⤴
	130	russian twisting taps	2	10	2–3	↻
	132	lunging rotating pass	2	10	2–3	↻
	120	push-ups (level 2)	2	5	2–3	⇄
	122	high pulls *	2	5	2–3	↑ ⤴ ⇄

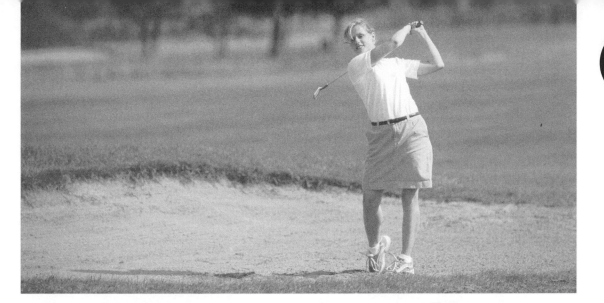

ADVANCED

	PAGE	EXERCISE	SETS	CONTACTS/ DISTANCE	RECOVERY (minutes)	GOAL
	99	tuck jumps	1	10	2–3	
	113	multiple hops over cones	2	10	2–3	
	103	standing lateral jump	2	10	2–3	
	118	box jump-ups	2	10	2–3	
	116	box jumps	2	10	2–3	
	117	depth jumps	2	5	2–3	
	125	wood chops	2	10	2–3	
	136	rotational slams	2	10	2–3	
	133	rotating pass on ball	2	10	2–3	
	123	hanging cleans *	2	5	2–3	

gymnastics

Gymnastics emphasizes linear speed and overall explosiveness, though floor exercises can require explosive changes of direction. Upper-body requisites are primarily push-pull in nature, though trunk rotation is also important in floor exercises, the pommel horse, and the vault. Before you jump into this program, start your plyometrics workout with the Dynamic Warm-Up & Muscle-Activation Series on pages 28–29.

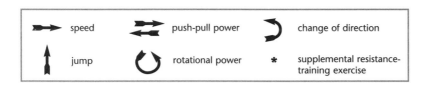

	speed		push-pull power		change of direction
	jump		rotational power	*	supplemental resistance-training exercise

	PAGE	EXERCISE	SETS	CONTACTS/ DISTANCE	RECOVERY (minutes)	GOAL
	102	standing broad jump	2	10	2–3	
	96	split jumps	2	10	2–3	
	101	squat jumps (1 leg)	2	10	2–3	
	114	speed skaters	2	10	2–3	
	124	tricep press pass	2	10	2–3	
	126	squat throws	2	10	2–3	
	120	push-ups	2	5	2–3	
	122	high pulls *	2	5	2–3	

INTERMEDIATE

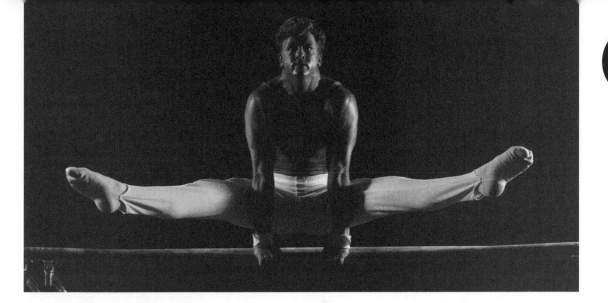

ADVANCED

	PAGE	EXERCISE	SETS	CONTACTS/ DISTANCE	RECOVERY (minutes)	GOAL
	99	tuck jumps	1	10	2–3	
	103	standing lateral jump	2	10	2–3	
	105	one-legged jumps	2	10	2–3	
	113	multiple hops over cones	2	10	2–3	
	116	box jumps	2	10	2–3	
	117	depth jumps	2	5	2–3	
	136	rotational slams	2	10	2–3	
	141	upper-body forward hops	2	10	2–3	
	133	rotating pass on ball	2	10	2–3	
	123	hanging cleans *	2	5	2–3	

ice/roller hockey

Hockey, be it on ice or roller skates, emphasizes sport-speed, or change of direction, as well as acceleration and first-step quickness. Upper-body requisites are primarily rotational power and explosiveness. Before you jump into this program, start your plyometrics workout with the Dynamic Warm-Up & Muscle-Activation Series on pages 28–29.

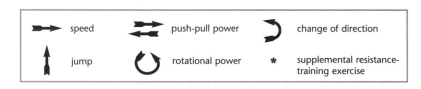

	speed		push-pull power		change of direction
	jump		rotational power	*	supplemental resistance-training exercise

INTERMEDIATE

	PAGE	EXERCISE	SETS	CONTACTS/DISTANCE	RECOVERY (minutes)	GOAL
	104	standing diagonal jump	2	10	2–3	↑ ⤴
	97	scissor jumps	2	10	2–3	➡ ↑
	112	slalom hops (1 leg)	2	10	2–3	↑ ⤴
	114	speed skaters	2	10	2–3	⤴
	129	pullover pass	2	10	2–3	⇄
	136	rotational slams	2	10	2–3	↻
	120	push-ups (level 2)	2	5	2–3	⇄
	122	high pulls *	2	5	2–3	➡ ↑ ⤴ ⇄

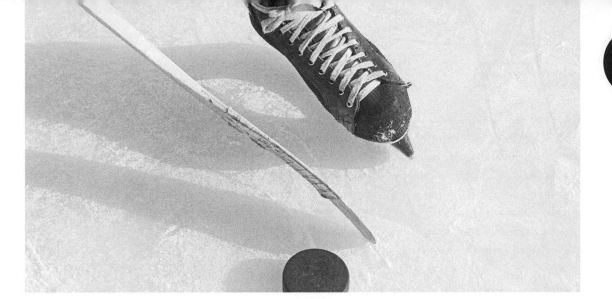

ADVANCED

	PAGE	EXERCISE	SETS	CONTACTS/ DISTANCE	RECOVERY (minutes)	GOAL
	99	tuck jumps	1	10	2–3	
	113	multiple hops over cones	2	10	2–3	
	103	standing lateral jump	2	10	2–3	
	105	one-legged jumps	2	10	2–3	
	116	box jumps	2	10	2–3	
	117	depth jumps	2	5	2–3	
	132	lunging rotating pass	2	10	2–3	
	137	vertical scoop toss	2	10	2–3	
	133	rotating pass on ball	2	10	2–3	
	123	hanging cleans *	2	5	2–3	

lacrosse

Lacrosse emphasizes sport-speed, or change of direction, but receivers and defensive backs need to focus on developing their linear speed. Upper-body requisites are primarily push-pull in nature, though explosive trunk rotation plays a big part in stick handling and offensive play. Before you jump into this program, start your plyometrics workout with the Dynamic Warm-Up & Muscle-Activation Series on pages 28–29.

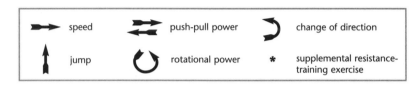

	speed		push-pull power		change of direction
	jump		rotational power	*	supplemental resistance-training exercise

INTERMEDIATE

	PAGE	EXERCISE	SETS	CONTACTS/DISTANCE	RECOVERY (minutes)	GOAL
	110	target hops	2	10	2–3	↑ ⤸
	111	target hops (1 leg)	2	10	2–3	↑ ⤸
	112	slalom hops (1 leg)	2	10	2–3	↑ ⤸
	114	speed skaters	2	10	2–3	⤸
	132	lunging rotating pass	2	10	2–3	↻
	139	back toss	2	10	2–3	↑ ⇄
	120	push-ups (level 2)	2	5	2–3	⇄
	122	high pulls *	2	5	2–3	→ ↑ ⤸ ⇄

ADVANCED

	PAGE	EXERCISE	SETS	CONTACTS/ DISTANCE	RECOVERY (minutes)	GOAL
	99	tuck jumps	1	10	2–3	
	113	multiple hops over cones	2	10	2–3	
	103	standing lateral jump	2	10	2–3	
	105	one-legged jumps	2	10	2–3	
	116	box jumps	2	10	2–3	
	117	depth jumps	2	5	2–3	
	125	wood chops	2	10	2–3	
	136	rotational slams	2	10	2–3	
	138	explosive start throws	2	10	2–3	
	123	hanging cleans *	2	5	2–3	

racquet sports

Both squash and racquetball emphasize sport-speed and first-step quickness. The upper body requires significant rotational power for quick pivoting and explosive trunk rotation when hitting the ball. Before you jump into this program, start your plyometrics workout with the Dynamic Warm-Up & Muscle-Activation Series on pages 28–29.

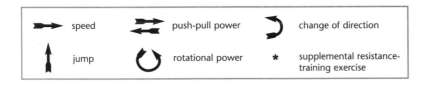

	speed		push-pull power		change of direction
	jump		rotational power	*	supplemental resistance-training exercise

INTERMEDIATE

	PAGE	EXERCISE	SETS	CONTACTS/ DISTANCE	RECOVERY (minutes)	GOAL
	106	90-degree jumps	2	10	2–3	
	97	scissor jumps	2	10	2–3	
	111	target hops (1 leg)	2	10	2–3	
	114	speed skaters	2	10	2–3	
	132	lunging rotating pass	2	10	2–3	
	126	squat throws	2	10	2–3	
	120	push-ups (level 2)	2	5	2–3	
	122	high pulls *	2	5	2–3	

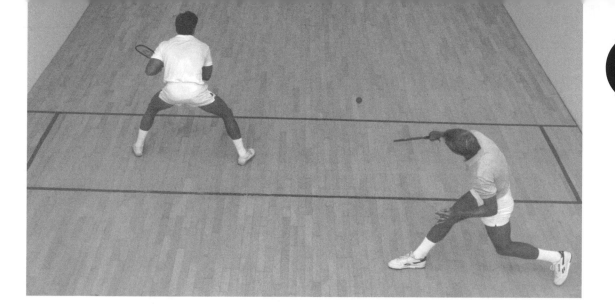

ADVANCED

	PAGE	EXERCISE	SETS	CONTACTS/ DISTANCE	RECOVERY (minutes)	GOAL
	118	box jump-ups	1	10	2–3	
	110	target hops	2	10	2–3	
	114	speed skaters	2	10	2–3	
	115	alternating straddle hops	2	10	2–3	
	116	box jumps	2	10	2–3	
	112	slalom hops (1 leg)	2	5	2–3	
	125	wood chops	2	10	2–3	
	136	rotational slams	2	10	2–3	
	138	explosive start throws	2	10	2–3	
	123	hanging cleans *	2	5	2–3	

rugby/australian football

Rugby and Australian football generally emphasize sport-speed, or change of direction, but wings and backs need to focus on developing their linear speed and explosiveness as well. Upper-body requisites are primarily push-pull in nature, though trunk rotation is important for ball handling and breakaway sprints. Before you jump into this program, start your plyometrics workout with the Dynamic Warm-Up & Muscle-Activation Series on pages 28–29.

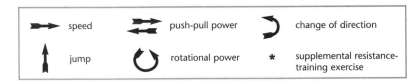

	speed		push-pull power		change of direction
	jump		rotational power	*	supplemental resistance-training exercise

INTERMEDIATE

	PAGE	EXERCISE	SETS	CONTACTS/ DISTANCE	RECOVERY (minutes)	GOAL
	102	standing broad jump	2	10	2–3	→ ↑ ⤸
	97	scissor jumps	2	10	2–3	→ ↑
	109	slalom hops	2	10	2–3	→ ↑ ⤸
	114	speed skaters	2	10	2–3	⤸
	127	chest pass	2	10	2–3	⇄
	126	squat throws	2	10	2–3	↑ ⇄
	120	push-ups (level 2)	2	5	2–3	⇄
	122	high pulls *	2	5	2–3	→ ↑ ⤸ ⇄

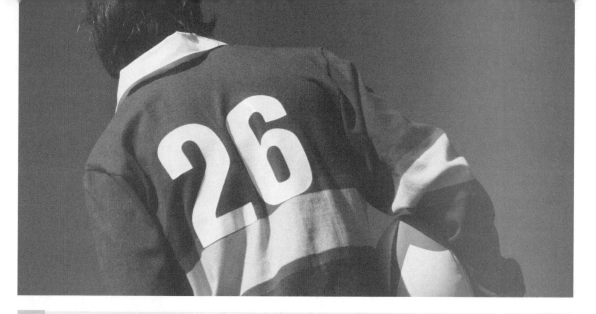

ADVANCED

	PAGE	EXERCISE	SETS	CONTACTS/ DISTANCE	RECOVERY (minutes)	GOAL
	99	tuck jumps	1	10	2–3	
	113	multiple hops over cones	2	10	2–3	
	103	standing lateral jump	2	10	2–3	
	105	one-legged jumps	2	10	2–3	
	116	box jumps	2	10	2–3	
	117	depth jumps	2	5	2–3	
	125	wood chops	2	10	2–3	
	136	rotational slams	2	10	2–3	
	137	vertical scoop toss	2	10	2–3	
	123	hanging cleans *	2	5	2–3	

skiing (alpine & nordic)

Alpine and Nordic skiing emphasize linear speed translated as power endurance in the linear plane. Upper-body requisites are primarily push-pull in nature, though trunk rotation is important for handling moguls and sudden turns on the slopes. Before you jump into this program, start your plyometrics workout with the Dynamic Warm-Up & Muscle-Activation Series on pages 28–29.

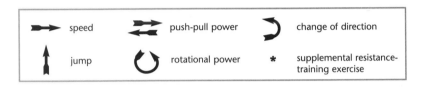

	speed		push-pull power		change of direction
	jump		rotational power	*	supplemental resistance-training exercise

INTERMEDIATE

	PAGE	EXERCISE	SETS	CONTACTS/DISTANCE	RECOVERY (minutes)	GOAL
	102	standing broad jump	2	10	2–3	
	109	slalom hops	2	10	2–3	
	114	speed skaters	2	10	2–3	
	101	squat jumps (1 leg)	2	10	2–3	
	129	pullover pass	2	10	2–3	
	126	squat throws	2	10	2–3	
	132	lunging rotating pass	2	5	2–3	
	122	high pulls *	2	5	2–3	

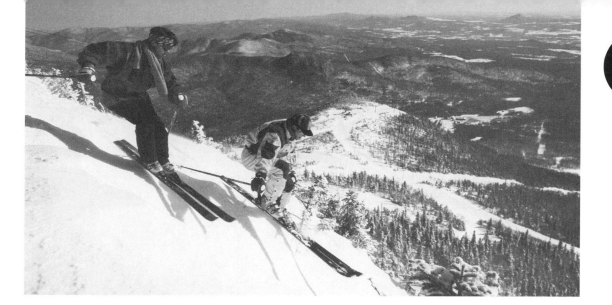

sking (alpine & nordic)

ADVANCED

	PAGE	EXERCISE	SETS	CONTACTS/ DISTANCE	RECOVERY (minutes)	GOAL
	99	tuck jumps	2	10	2–3	
	113	multiple hops over cones	2	10	2–3	
	103	standing lateral jump	2	10	2–3	
	105	one-legged jumps	2	10	2–3	
	116	box jumps	2	10	2–3	
	117	depth jumps	2	5	2–3	
	125	wood chops	2	10	2–3	
	136	rotational slams	2	10	2–3	
	139	back toss	2	10	2–3	
	123	hanging cleans *	2	5	2–3	

soccer

Soccer places a great emphasis on sport-speed, or change of direction, though the occasional breakaway will require significant acceleration. Goal keepers should work on explosiveness, push-pull power, and first-step quickness. Before you jump into this program, start your plyometrics workout with the Dynamic Warm-Up & Muscle-Activation Series on pages 28–29.

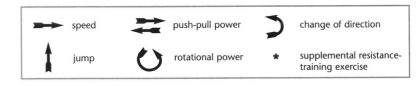

speed • push-pull power • change of direction • jump • rotational power • * supplemental resistance-training exercise

INTERMEDIATE

	PAGE	EXERCISE	SETS	CONTACTS/DISTANCE	RECOVERY (minutes)	GOAL
	110	target hops	2	10	2–3	↑⤵
	111	target hops (1 leg)	2	10	2–3	↑⤵
	112	slalom hops (1 leg)	2	10	2–3	↑⤵
	114	speed skaters	2	10	2–3	⤵
	132	lunging rotating pass	2	10	2–3	↻
	139	back toss	2	10	2–3	↑ ⇄
	120	push-ups (level 2)	2	5	2–3	⇄
	122	high pulls *	2	5	2–3	→ ↑⤵ ⇄

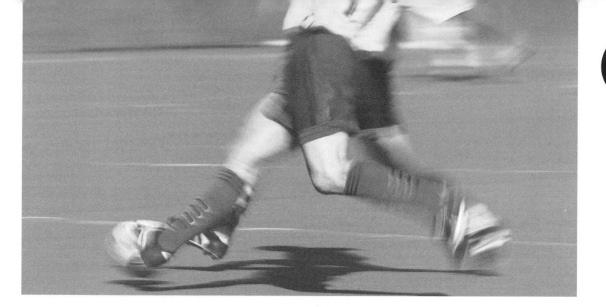

ADVANCED

	PAGE	EXERCISE	SETS	CONTACTS/ DISTANCE	RECOVERY (minutes)	GOAL
	99	tuck jumps	1	10	2–3	
	113	multiple hops over cones	2	10	2–3	
	103	standing lateral jump	2	10	2–3	
	105	one-legged jumps	2	10	2–3	
	116	box jumps	2	10	2–3	
	117	depth jumps	2	5	2–3	
	125	wood chops	2	10	2–3	
	136	rotational slams	2	10	2–3	
	138	explosive start throws	2	10	2–3	
	123	hanging cleans *	2	5	2–3	

swimming

Swimming requires a tremendous amount of push-pull power, primarily in the upper body. A powerful core, however, is necessary to utilize the upper body efficiently in the water, regardless of stroke, so rotational power should also be emphasized during upper-body training. The butterfly stroke places an emphasis on lower-body power in the linear plane, so linear-speed exercises will help. Before you jump into this program, start your plyometrics workout with the Dynamic Warm-Up & Muscle-Activation Series on pages 28–29.

➡ speed	⇄ push-pull power	↪ change of direction
↑ jump	↻ rotational power	* supplemental resistance-training exercise

INTERMEDIATE

	PAGE	EXERCISE	SETS	CONTACTS/DISTANCE	RECOVERY (minutes)	GOAL
	102	standing broad jump	2	10	2–3	➡ ↑ ↪
	97	scissor jumps	2	10	2–3	➡ ↑
	114	speed skaters	2	10	2–3	↪
	96	split jumps	2	10	2–3	➡ ↑
	125	wood chops	2	10	2–3	↑ ⇄
	132	lunging rotating pass	2	10	2–3	↻
	129	pullover pass	2	5	2–3	⇄
	122	high pulls *	2	5	2–3	➡ ↑ ↪ ⇄

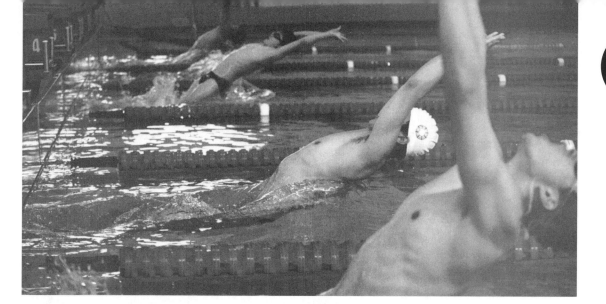

ADVANCED

	PAGE	EXERCISE	SETS	CONTACTS/DISTANCE	RECOVERY (minutes)	GOAL
	99	tuck jumps	1	10	2–3	
	113	multiple hops over cones	2	10	2–3	
	102	standing broad jump	2	10	2–3	
	116	box jumps	2	10	2–3	
	117	depth jumps	2	5	2–3	
	125	wood chops	2	10	2–3	
	136	rotational slams	2	10	2–3	
	139	back toss	2	10	2–3	
	133	rotating pass on ball	2	10	2–3	
	123	hanging cleans *	2	5	2–3	

tennis

Tennis emphasizes sport-speed, and first-step quickness. The tennis player's upper body requires significant rotational power for quick pivoting and explosive trunk rotation when hitting the ball. Before you jump into this program, start your plyometrics workout with the Dynamic Warm-Up & Muscle-Activation Series on pages 28–29.

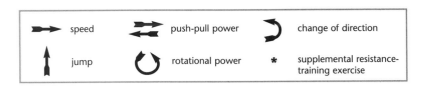

	speed		push-pull power		change of direction
	jump		rotational power	*	supplemental resistance-training exercise

INTERMEDIATE

	PAGE	EXERCISE	SETS	CONTACTS/ DISTANCE	RECOVERY (minutes)	GOAL
	106	90-degree jumps	2	10	2–3	
	97	scissor jumps	2	10	2–3	
	111	target hops (1 leg)	2	10	2–3	
	114	speed skaters	2	10	2–3	
	128	overhead pass	2	10	2–3	
	131	standing rotating pass	2	10	2–3	
	120	push-ups (level 2)	2	5	2–3	
	122	high pulls *	2	5	2–3	

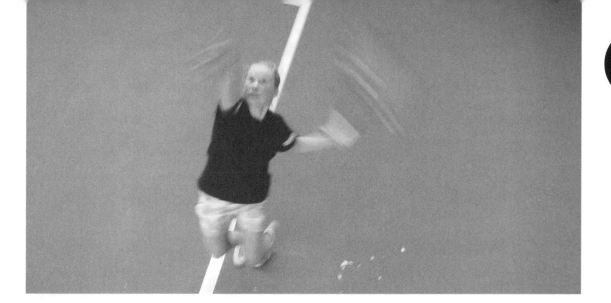

ADVANCED

	PAGE	EXERCISE	SETS	CONTACTS/ DISTANCE	RECOVERY (minutes)	GOAL
	118	box jump-ups	1	10	2–3	
	99	tuck jumps	2	10	2–3	
	113	multiple hops over cones	2	10	2–3	
	110	target hops	2	10	2–3	
	116	box jumps	2	10	2–3	
	117	depth jumps	2	5	2–3	
	125	wood chops	2	10	2–3	
	136	rotational slams	2	10	2–3	
	138	explosive start throws	2	10	2–3	
	123	hanging cleans *	2	5	2–3	

track & field—jumping events

Jumping events in track and field emphasize linear speed and overall explosiveness. Upperbody requisites are primarily push-pull in nature, though trunk rotation is important in sprinting, which often precedes the actual jump in the event. Before you jump into this program, start your plyometrics workout with the Dynamic Warm-Up & Muscle-Activation Series on pages 28–29.

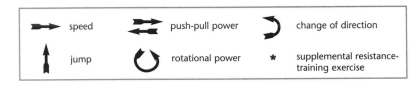

| ➤ | speed | ⇄ | push-pull power | ↪ | change of direction |
| ↑ | jump | ↻ | rotational power | * | supplemental resistance-training exercise |

INTERMEDIATE

	PAGE	EXERCISE	SETS	CONTACTS/ DISTANCE	RECOVERY (minutes)	GOAL
	102	standing broad jump	2	10	2–3	➤ ↑ ↪
	96	split jumps	2	10	2–3	➤ ↑
	110	target hops	2	10	2–3	↑ ↪
	114	speed skaters	2	10	2–3	↪
	137	vertical scoop toss	2	10	2–3	↑ ⇄
	125	wood chops	2	10	2–3	↑ ⇄
	120	push-ups (level 2)	2	5	2–3	⇄
	122	high pulls *	2	5	2–3	➤ ↑ ↪ ⇄

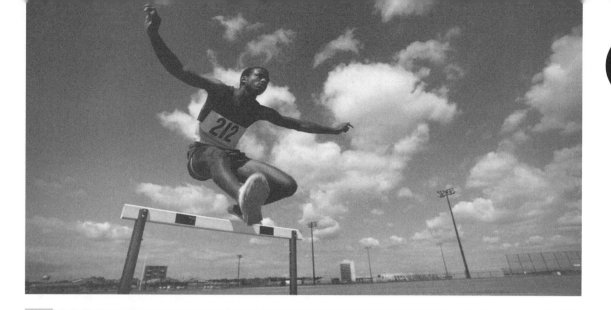

ADVANCED

	PAGE	EXERCISE	SETS	CONTACTS/DISTANCE	RECOVERY (minutes)	GOAL
	99	tuck jumps	1	10	2–3	
	113	multiple hops over cones	2	10	2–3	
	103	standing lateral jump	2	10	2–3	
	105	one-legged jumps	2	10	2–3	
	116	box jumps	2	10	2–3	
	117	depth jumps	2	5	2–3	
	139	back toss	2	10	2–3	
	136	rotational slams	2	10	2–3	
	138	explosive start throws	2	10	2–3	
	123	hanging cleans *	2	5	2–3	

track & field—running events

Running events in track and field place a huge emphasis on linear speed, both for acceleration and maximum velocity. Upper-body requisites are primarily push-pull in nature, though trunk rotation is important in sprinting, for both power and running efficiency. Before you jump into this program, start your plyometrics workout with the Dynamic Warm-Up & Muscle-Activation Series on pages 28–29.

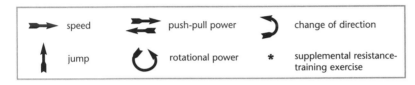

	speed		push-pull power		change of direction
	jump		rotational power	*	supplemental resistance-training exercise

INTERMEDIATE

	PAGE	EXERCISE	SETS	CONTACTS/DISTANCE	RECOVERY (minutes)	GOAL
	102	standing broad jump	2	10	2–3	speed jump change of direction
	96	split jumps	2	10	2–3	speed jump
	101	squat jumps (1 leg)	2	10	2–3	speed jump change of direction
	114	speed skaters	2	10	2–3	change of direction
	132	lunging rotating pass	2	10	2–3	rotational power
	125	wood chops	2	10	2–3	jump push-pull power
	120	push-ups (level 2)	2	5	2–3	push-pull power
	122	high pulls *	2	5	2–3	speed jump change of direction push-pull power

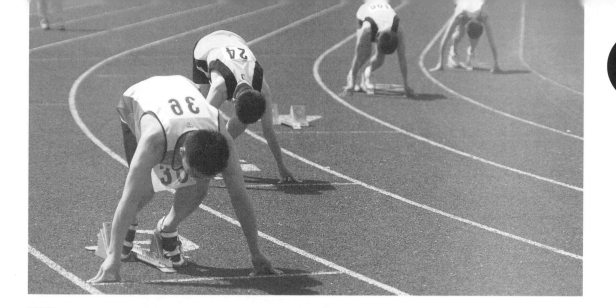

ADVANCED

	PAGE	EXERCISE	SETS	CONTACTS / DISTANCE	RECOVERY (minutes)	GOAL
	99	tuck jumps	1	10	2–3	
	113	multiple hops over cones	2	10	2–3	
	98	split jumps w/cycle	2	10	2–3	
	105	one-legged jumps	2	10	2–3	
	116	box jumps	2	10	2–3	
	117	depth jumps	2	5	2–3	
	125	wood chops	2	10	2–3	
	136	rotational slams	2	10	2–3	
	138	explosive start throws	2	10	2–3	
	123	hanging cleans *	2	5	2–3	

track & field—throwing events

Throwing events in track and field emphasize single-repetition explosiveness. Trunk rotation plays a huge part in all throwing events regardless of event or throwing style, so rotational power should be the training focus. Before you jump into this program, start your plyometrics workout with the Dynamic Warm-Up & Muscle-Activation Series on pages 28–29.

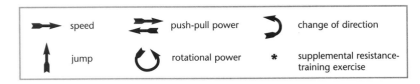

		speed		push-pull power		change of direction
		jump		rotational power	*	supplemental resistance-training exercise

INTERMEDIATE

	PAGE	EXERCISE	SETS	CONTACTS/DISTANCE	RECOVERY (minutes)	GOAL
	102	standing broad jump	2	10	2–3	
	97	scissor jumps	2	10	2–3	
	109	slalom hops	2	10	2–3	
	114	speed skaters	2	10	2–3	
	136	rotational slams	2	10	2–3	
	126	squat throws	2	10	2–3	
	120	push-ups (level 2)	2	5	2–3	
	122	high pulls *	2	5	2–3	

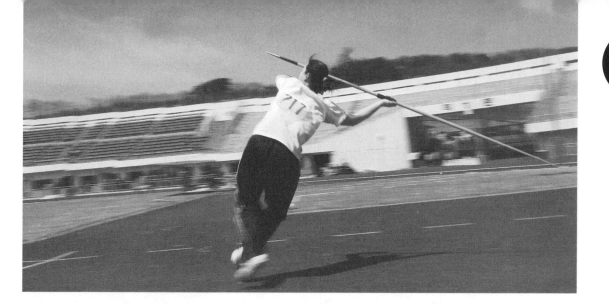

ADVANCED

	PAGE	EXERCISE	SETS	CONTACTS/ DISTANCE	RECOVERY (minutes)	GOAL
	99	tuck jumps	1	10	2–3	
	113	multiple hops over cones	2	10	2–3	
	103	standing lateral jump	2	10	2–3	
	105	one-legged jumps	2	10	2–3	
	116	box jumps	2	10	2–3	
	117	depth jumps	2	5	2–3	
	125	wood chops	2	10	2–3	
	137	vertical scoop toss	2	10	2–3	
	141	upper-body forward hops	2	10	2–3	
	123	hanging cleans *	2	5	2–3	

volleyball

Volleyball emphasizes sport-speed, but first-step quickness and jumping power are crucial. Upper-body requisites are primarily push-pull in nature for the offensive player, while explosive trunk rotation plays a big part for the defensive player. Before you jump into this program, start your plyometrics workout with the Dynamic Warm-Up & Muscle-Activation Series on pages 28–29.

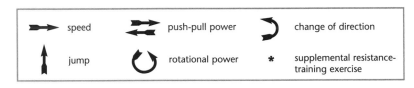

		speed			push-pull power			change of direction
		jump			rotational power	*		supplemental resistance-training exercise

INTERMEDIATE

	PAGE	EXERCISE	SETS	CONTACTS/DISTANCE	RECOVERY (minutes)	GOAL
	95	squat jumps	2	10	2–3	➤ ↑ ↺
	97	scissor jumps	2	10	2–3	➤ ↑
	109	slalom hops	2	10	2–3	➤ ↑ ↺
	114	speed skaters	2	10	2–3	↺
	137	vertical scoop toss	2	10	2–3	↑ ⇄
	136	rotational slams	2	10	2–3	↻
	134	medicine ball slams	2	5	2–3	↑ ⇄
	122	high pulls *	2	5	2–3	➤ ↑ ↺ ⇄

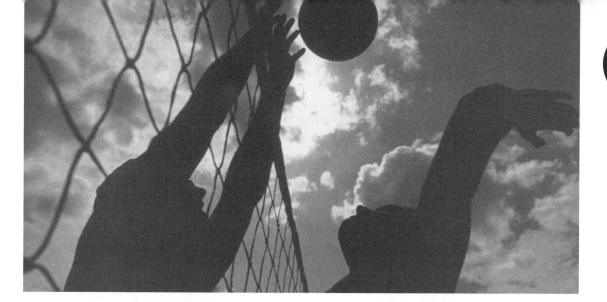

ADVANCED

	PAGE	EXERCISE	SETS	CONTACTS/ DISTANCE	RECOVERY (minutes)	GOAL
	99	tuck jumps	1	10	2–3	
	113	multiple hops over cones	2	10	2–3	
	106	90-degree jumps	2	10	2–3	
	105	one-legged jumps	2	10	2–3	
	116	box jumps	2	10	2–3	
	117	depth jumps	2	5	2–3	
	125	wood chops	2	10	2–3	
	139	back toss	2	10	2–3	
	141	upper-body forward hops	2	10	2–3	
	123	hanging cleans *	2	5	2–3	

wrestling

Wrestling emphasizes acceleration and first-step quickness. The upper-body requisite is primarily for massive amounts of rotational power and explosiveness, though push-pull power can also come in handy for the offensive wrestler. Before you jump into this program, start your plyometrics workout with the Dynamic Warm-Up & Muscle-Activation Series on pages 28–29.

	speed		push-pull power		change of direction
	jump		rotational power	*	supplemental resistance-training exercise

INTERMEDIATE

	PAGE	EXERCISE	SETS	CONTACTS/DISTANCE	RECOVERY (minutes)	GOAL
	102	standing broad jump	2	10	2–3	
	100	counter-movement jumps, 1-leg	2	10	2–3	
	114	speed skaters	2	10	2–3	
	129	pullover pass	2	10	1–2	
	126	squat throws	2	10	1–2	
	136	rotational slams	2	10	1–2	
	135	shot put	2	5	2–3	
	122	high pulls *	2	5	2–3	

ADVANCED

	PAGE	EXERCISE	SETS	CONTACTS/ DISTANCE	RECOVERY (minutes)	GOAL
	99	tuck jumps	1	10	2–3	
	113	multiple hops over cones	2	10	2–3	
	103	standing lateral jump	2	10	2–3	
	116	box jumps	2	10	2–3	
	117	depth jumps	2	5	2–3	
	139	back toss	2	10	1–2	
	133	rotating pass on ball	2	10	1–2	
	137	vertical scoop toss	2	10	1–2	
	140	push "over the top"	2	10	1–2	
	141	upper-body forward hops	2	10	1–2	
	123	hanging cleans *	2	5	2–3	

part three:

the
exercises

forward skips

Speed

Jump

COD

STARTING POSITION: Stand with your left foot forward. Your right arm is forward and left arm is back, both elbows bent about 90 degrees.

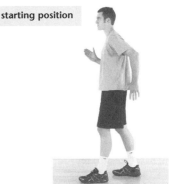

starting position

1 Driving off your left leg, pushing in the down and backward direction, drive your right knee forward and upward and your right elbow backward as your left elbow moves forward. Your goal is to attain vertical lift. Maintain an erect posture and focus on keeping your ankles flexed.

2 Driving off your right leg, pushing in the down and backward direction, drive your left knee forward and upward and your left elbow backward. Make sure your arms and legs are synchronized on every skip.

Repeat, alternating legs.

BENEFIT

Actively warms up the body; applies horizontal force into the ground for vertical lift. This is crucial to any athlete involved in sprinting or forward jumping–related sports.

Speed

Jump

COD

STARTING POSITION: Stand with your feet wider than your shoulders. Place your hands lightly behind your head.

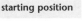
starting position

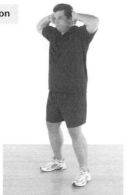

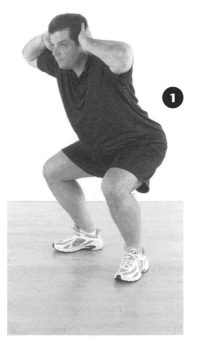

1

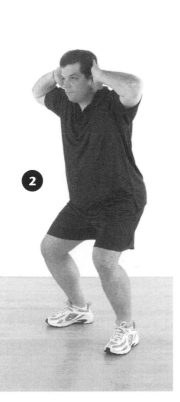

2

1 Sit back by bending at the knees, keeping your back as straight as possible and shins vertical. Your weight should be on your heels; be sure not to shift forward.

2 Return to starting position.

Repeat.

BENEFIT

Actively warms up the deep hip muscles, the quadriceps and the hamstrings; activates the core stabilizers of the spine. Maintaining core stability is crucial to any athlete regardless of their sport.

Speed

Jump

COD

STARTING POSITION: Stand with your left foot forward. Your right arm is forward and left arm is back, both elbows bent about 90 degrees.

starting position

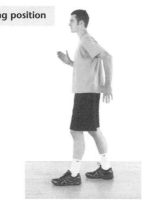

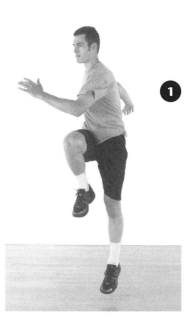

1

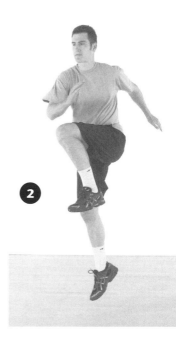

2

1 Driving off your left leg, pushing in the down and backward direction, lift your right knee upward and laterally, making a circle from right to center. Allow your arms to move freely.

2 Land your right foot directly under your right hip in a flat-footed position and immediately drive your right foot down and back, lifting your left knee upward and laterally, making a circle from left to center.

Repeat, alternating sides.

BENEFIT

Actively warms up the deep internal rotators of the hip, the hip flexors and the hamstrings; activates the dynamic stabilizers of the spine. These are very important attributes to any athlete who needs to change direction quickly and explosively.

dynamic warm-up
alternating side squats
level I

77

Speed

Jump

COD

STARTING POSITION: Stand with your feet together and hands on your hips.

starting position

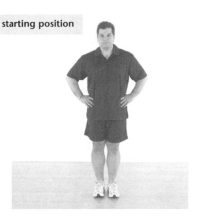

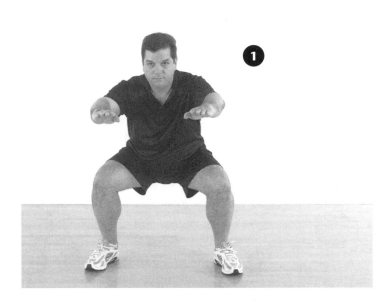

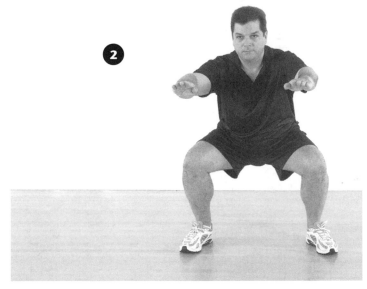

1 Step to the right, bending down into a parallel squat position while maintaining a straight back. Keep your arms out in front of you to help you maintain balance.

2 Return to starting position and repeat to the left side.

Repeat, alternating sides.

BENEFIT

Actively warms up the deep adductors of the hip, the quadriceps and the hamstrings; activates the core stabilizers of the spine. Maintaining core stability is crucial to any athlete regardless of their sport.

Speed

Jump

COD

STARTING POSITION: Stand with your feet together and your arms at your sides, both elbows bent about 90 degrees.

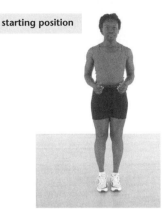

starting position

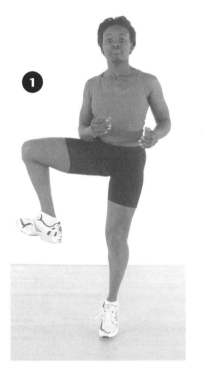

1

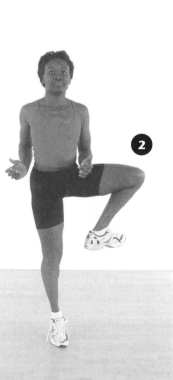

2

1 Driving off your left leg, pushing in the down and forward direction, lift your right knee upward, circling from center to right. Allow your arms to move freely to help you maintain balance throughout the exercise.

2 Land your right foot directly under your right hip in a flat-footed position and immediately drive your right foot down and back, lifting your left knee upward, circling from center to left.

Repeat, alternating sides.

BENEFIT

Actively warms up the deep external rotators of the hip, the hip flexors and the quadriceps; activates the dynamic stabilizers of the spine. These are very important attributes for any athlete who needs to backpedal, or step back and change direction quickly and explosively.

Speed

Jump

COD

STARTING POSITION: Stand with your feet together, arms at your sides.

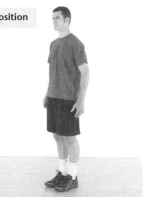

starting position

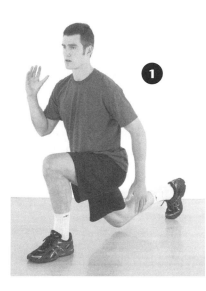

1

1 Step back onto the ball of your right foot into a lunging position, keeping your right knee slightly bent and your left foot flat on the ground. You can use your arms for balance. Keep your back straight and head up.

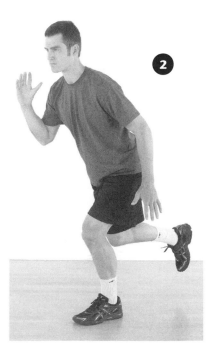

2

2 Drive your left heel into the ground to raise your pelvis and return your right foot to starting position.

Repeat, alternating sides.

BENEFIT

Actively warms up the hip extensors, quadriceps and hamstrings; activates the core stabilizers of the spine. Maintaining core stability is crucial to any athlete regardless of their sport.

Speed

Jump

COD

STARTING POSITION: Stand in the athletic ready position, with knees slightly bent, back flat, and shoulders in front of hips.

starting position

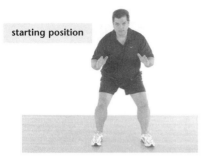

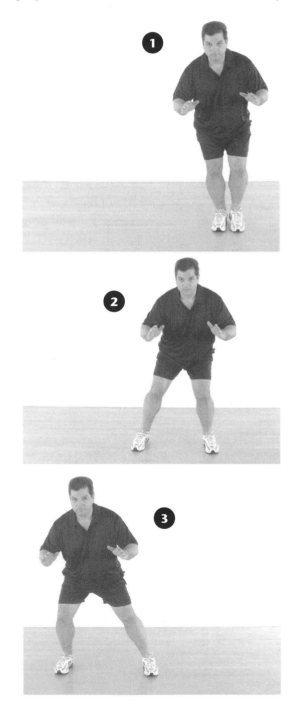

1 Pull with your right leg as you step with your left foot, bringing your feet together. Do not cross your feet when shuffling and keep a wide base at all times. Always have one foot in contact with the ground when practicing this drill.

2 Push off with your left leg as you step to the right and plant your right foot. Keep both feet pointed straight ahead in the direction you are facing. Focus on keeping your hips and head level; move directly to the side without "bouncing" up and down.

3 Step your right foot next to your left, then push off with your right leg as you step to the left.

Repeat, alternating sides.

BENEFIT

Actively warms up the abductors and adductors; improves lateral movement skill ability.

Speed

Jump

COD

This is an ideal Change of Direction exercise.

STARTING POSITION: Stand with your feet together.

starting position

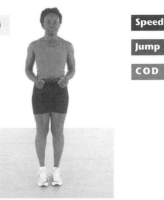

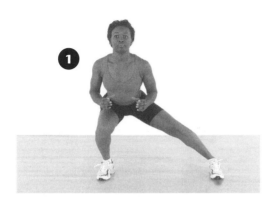

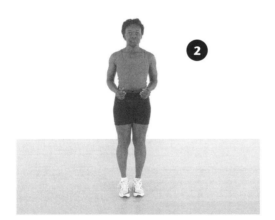

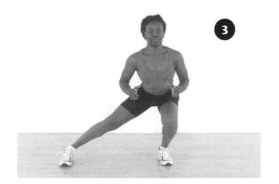

1 Maintaining a straight back and keeping your hands forward in an athletic ready position, lunge wide to the right and "sit down" on your right hip. Align the nose, knee and toe.

2 Drive your right heel into the ground to return to starting position.

3 Repeat to the left side. Always keep your feet facing forward, stepping directly to the side.

Repeat, alternating sides.

BENEFIT

Actively warms up the hip adductors, rotators, and gluteal muscles; activates the core stabilizers of the spine. Maintaining core stability is crucial to any athlete regardless of their sport.

82

Speed

Jump

COD

STARTING POSITION: Stand in the athletic ready position, with knees slightly bent, back flat and shoulders in front of hips.

starting position

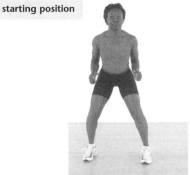

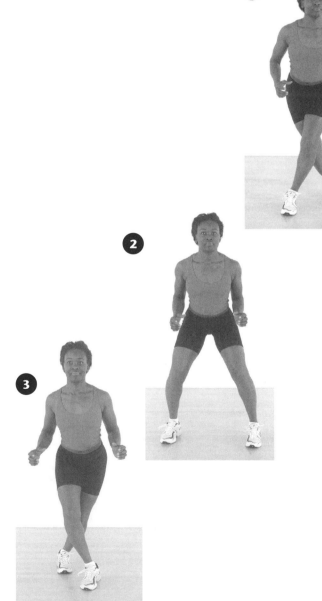

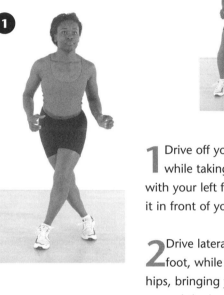

1 Drive off your right foot while taking a crossover step with your left foot and planting it in front of your body.

2 Drive laterally off your left foot, while rotating your hips, bringing your right foot around the back of your body and planting it directly to the right of your body.

3 Drive off your right foot while rotating your hips and bringing your left foot around the back of your body.

Repeat, alternating stepping across the front of your body and then around the back.

BENEFIT

Actively warms up the body; enhances pelvic and trunk mobility.

level I

83

STARTING POSITION: From the athletic ready position, lower your hips slightly into a half-squat position while keeping your back straight.

starting position

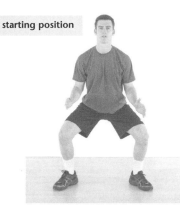

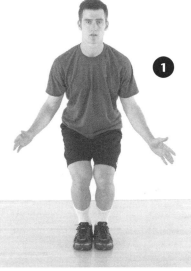

1 Quickly and simultaneously jump your feet together, keeping your knees bent at all times and not lifting your feet too far off the floor.

2 Maintaining the half-squat position, jump both feet apart and open the legs so that the knees and toes point to the sides. Stay low!

Jump your feet back together and repeat.

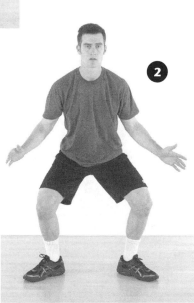

BENEFIT

Actively warms up the gluteal muscles, internal and external hip rotators, and quadriceps.

backward cycle run

84

Speed

Jump

COD

This drill requires enough space in which to move backward.

STARTING POSITION: Stand with your feet together. You will be moving backward in this exercise, creating a backward "cycling" motion with your legs.

starting position

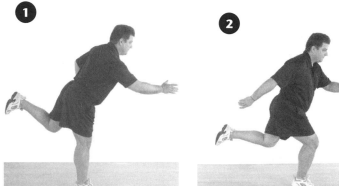

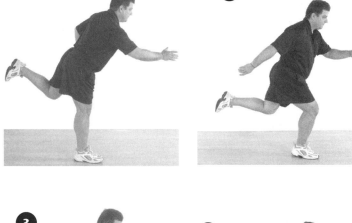

1–2 Keeping your left ankle flexed, bring your left heel to your butt and explosively leap backward off the ball of your right foot while extending your left leg to reach back to land on the ball of your left foot.

3–4 As you land on your left foot, fire your right heel to your butt and explosively leap backward off your left foot while extending your right leg to reach back to land on your right foot.

Repeat, alternating legs.

BENEFIT

Actively warms up and develops dynamic flexibility of the hip flexors.

STARTING POSITION: Lie flat on your back with your arms at your sides, palms flat on the ground and legs straight.

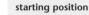

starting position

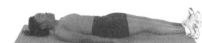

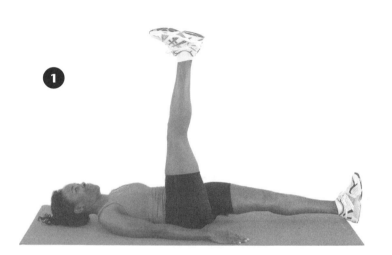

1 Keeping your abdominals tight, your ankles flexed and your legs fairly straight, explosively lift your right leg up toward your chest.

2 At the height of the lift, immediately lower your right leg back to the ground. Maintain control throughout the movement so that your foot does not crash onto the floor when you lower it, and keep your abdominals tight and the opposite leg flat on the ground.

Repeat, then switch legs.

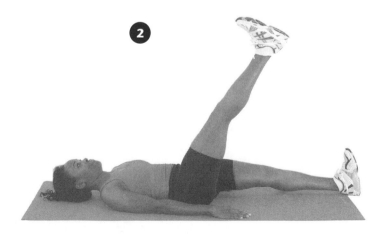

BENEFIT

Enhances mobilization of the hip flexors, as well as dynamic flexibility of the hip extensors.

lateral leg raises

Speed

Jump

COD

STARTING POSITION: Lie on your right side in a straight line, aligning your shoulders, hips and ankles. Keep your abdominals tight, both ankles flexed and your top foot slightly pointed down (internally rotated at the hip).

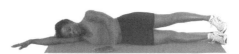

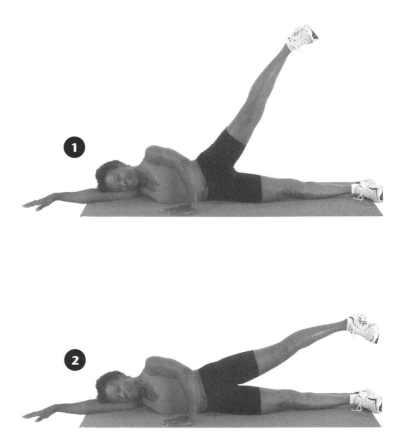

1 Explosively lift your left leg up toward the ceiling.

2 At the height of the lift, immediately lower your left leg back to the ground. Maintain control throughout the movement so that your foot does not crash onto the opposite leg when you lower it.

Repeat, then lie on your left side and repeat with your right leg.

BENEFIT

Enhances mobilization of the hip abductors, as well as dynamic flexibility of the hip adductors.

STARTING POSITION: Lie on your left side with your left leg straight and flexed at the ankle and the foot of your right leg placed flat on the floor at hip height. You may grab your right ankle with your right hand to stabilize in this position.

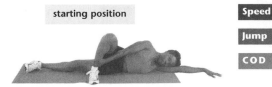

starting position

Speed

Jump

COD

1 Explosively lift your left thigh off the ground while keeping your left foot parallel to the ground.

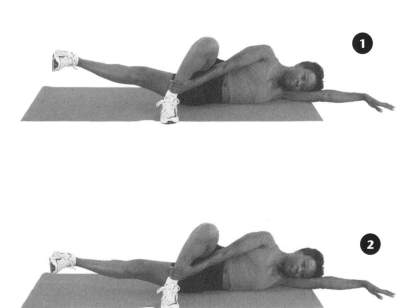

1

2 At the height of the lift, immediately lower your left leg back to the ground. Maintain control throughout the movement so that your foot does not crash onto the floor when you lower it.

2

Repeat, then lie on your right side and repeat with your right leg.

BENEFIT

Enhances mobilization of the hip adductors, as well as dynamic flexibility of the hip abductors.

Speed

Jump

COD

STARTING POSITION: Begin in quadruped position, with your hands directly under your shoulders and knees directly under your hips. Your shoulders and hips must stay square and parallel to the ground without any bending of the elbows or leaning to one side throughout the entire movement.

starting position

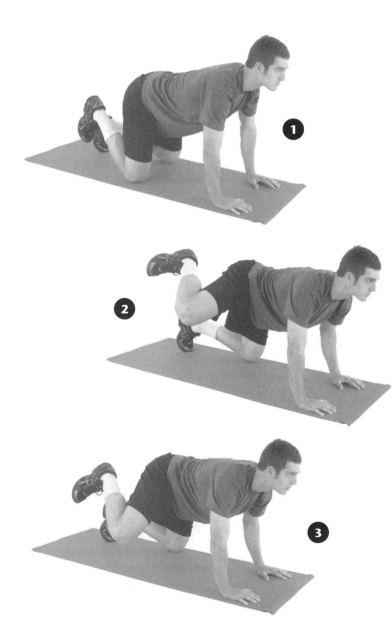

1 Bend your right knee so that your calf is touching your hamstring. Keep both ankles flexed throughout this movement.

2 Keeping the calf/hamstring contact, explosively lift your right leg diagonally backward at a 45-degree angle. Do not lift your hip up as you lift your knee off the ground.

3 At the height of the movement, return your right knee to starting position. Maintain control throughout this exercise so that you do not slam your knee on the ground on the way down.

Repeat, then switch legs.

BENEFIT

Enhances mobilization of the external hip rotators, as well as dynamic flexibility of the internal hip rotators.

Speed

Jump

COD

STARTING POSITION: Begin in quadruped position, with your hands directly under your shoulders and knees directly under your hips. Your shoulders and hips must stay square and parallel to the ground without any bending of the elbows or leaning to one side throughout the entire movement.

starting position

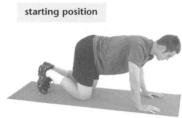

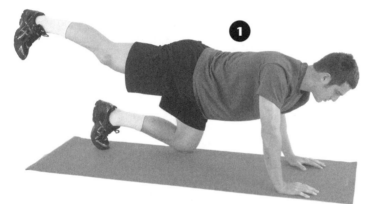

1 Explosively extend and straighten your right leg back.

2 Immediately upon straightening the right leg back, bend your knee, lifting it to the side while rotating the right hip joint in a counter-clockwise direction. Picture your right knee making large forward circles during this movement. Maintain control throughout this exercise, keeping a stable quadruped position.

Repeat, then switch legs.

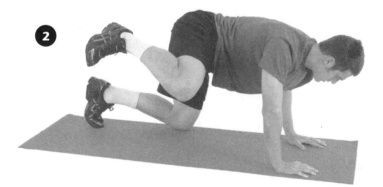

BENEFIT

Enhances mobilization and dynamic flexibility of the external and internal rotators of the hip.

Speed

Jump

COD

STARTING POSITION: Begin in quadruped position, with your hands directly under your shoulders and knees directly under your hips. Your shoulders and hips must stay square and parallel to the ground without any bending of the elbows or leaning to one side throughout the entire movement.

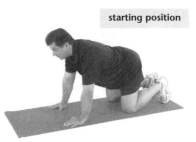

starting position

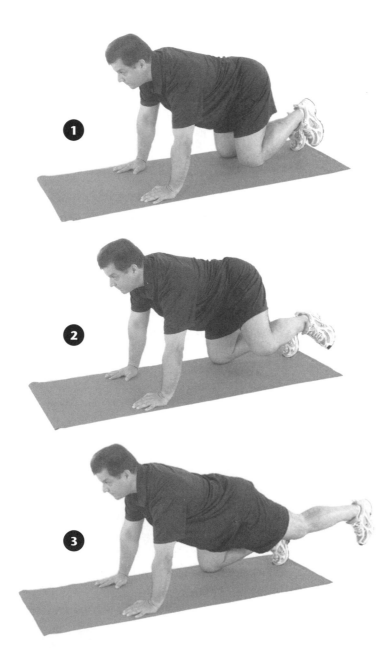

1 Bend your left knee so that your calf is touching your hamstring.

2 Maintaining the calf/hamstring contact, explosively lift your left leg to the side.

3 Immediately upon reaching the height of the lift, extend your left leg back, straightening your leg while rotating your right hip joint in a clockwise direction. Picture your left knee making large backward circles during this movement. Maintain control throughout this exercise, keeping a stable quadruped position.

Repeat, then switch legs.

BENEFIT

Enhances mobilization and dynamic flexibility of the internal and external rotators of the hip.

STARTING POSITION: Begin in quadruped position, with your hands directly under your shoulders and knees directly under your hips. Your shoulders and hips must stay square and parallel to the ground without any bending of the elbows or leaning to one side throughout the entire movement.

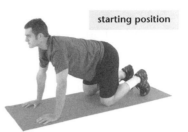

starting position

Speed

Jump

COD

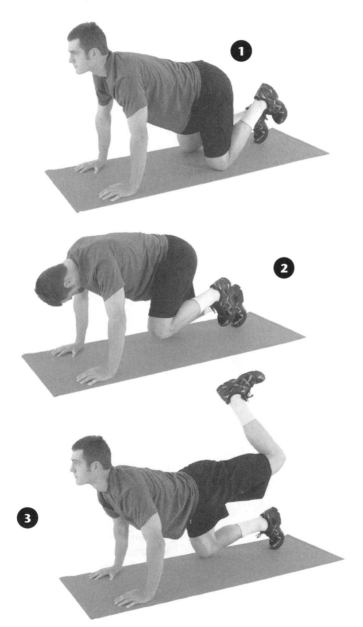

1 Bend your left knee so that your calf is touching your hamstring. Keep both ankles flexed throughout this movement.

2 Keeping the calf/hamstring contact, flex your thigh and drop your chin as you bring your knee to your chest.

3 Extend your left thigh, back and neck, arching back with your left leg and keeping your ankle flexed. Envision trying to touch your heel to your head.

Repeat, then switch legs.

BENEFIT

Enhances mobilization and dynamic flexibility of the flexors and extensors of the hip.

seated hip thrusts

level I

STARTING POSITION: Sit on the ground with your legs extended in front of you and your ankles flexed. Place your hands on the ground behind your hips with your fingers pointed toward your feet.

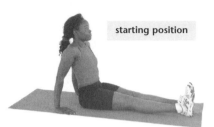

starting position

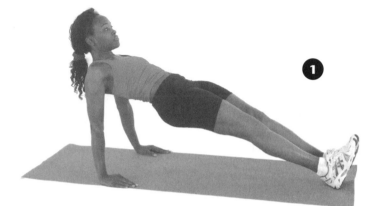

1

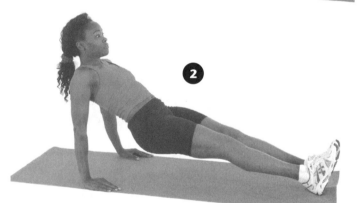

2

1 Push your heels into the ground and, with your arms extended and supporting your weight on your hands, raise your hips as high as possible into a hyperextension position.

2–3 Lower your hips back to starting position and quickly and explosively pop them back up.

Repeat.

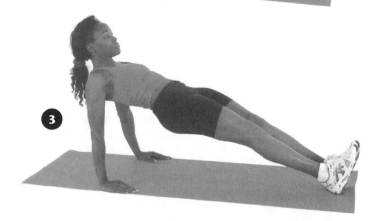

3

BENEFIT

Enhances mobilization and power development of the hip extensors.

STARTING POSITION: Sit on the ground with your legs extended in front of you and your ankles flexed. Place your hands on the ground behind your hips with your fingers pointed toward your feet.

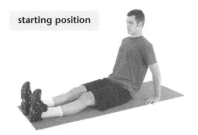

starting position

Speed

Jump

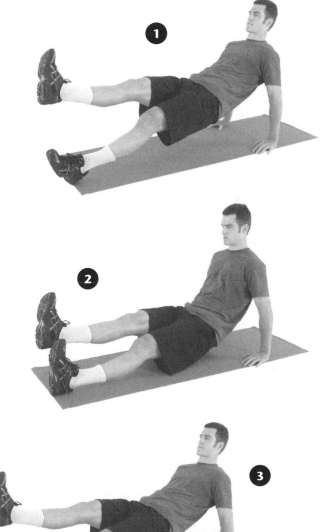

1 Raise and hold your right leg totally off the ground. Pushing your left heel into the ground, with your arms extended and supporting your weight on your hands, raise your hips as high as possible into a hyperextension position.

2–3 Lower your hips back to starting position and quickly and explosively pop them back up.

Repeat, then switch legs.

BENEFIT

Enhances mobilization and power development of the hip extensors.

Speed

Jump

COD

STARTING POSITION: Stand with your feet hip-width apart and your arms at your sides.

starting position

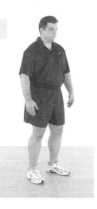

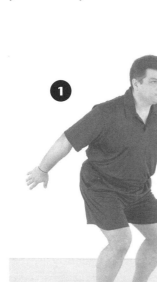

1

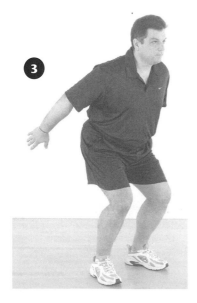

3

2

1 Keeping your weight on your heels, quickly lower your hips into a quarter-squat, pushing them back while flexing your knees. As this happens, swing your arms backward.

2 Without pausing, reverse direction explosively and jump straight up into the air.

3 When landing, make sure that you absorb the impact by pushing your hips back and flexing your knees.

Repeat.

BENEFIT

Actively warms up and develops dynamic flexibility of the hip flexors.

STARTING POSITION: Stand with your feet hip-width apart and your hands at your sides or clasped behind your head.

Speed

Jump

COD

starting position

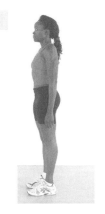

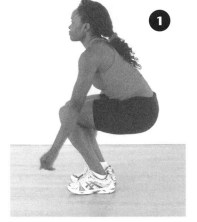

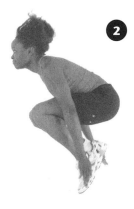

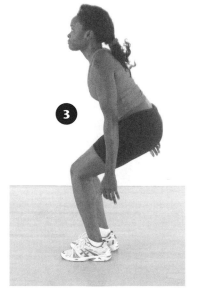

1 Keeping your weight on your heels, squat down until your thighs are parallel to the floor. Pause in the squat.

2 Without counter-movement and without the use of your arms, jump as high as possible.

3 When landing, make sure to absorb the impact by pushing your hips back and flexing your knees.

Repeat.

BENEFIT

Develops overall power and enhances the lower body's ability to decelerate.

split jumps

level II

Speed
Jump

This is a high-intensity plyometric exercise that is suitable only for intermediate-to-advanced athletes. You should be familiar with lunges before attempting this.

STARTING POSITION: From standing, step your left foot back into a lunge stance, keeping your right knee bent. Contract your abdominal muscles to stabilize your trunk and spine.

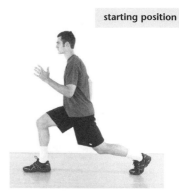

starting position

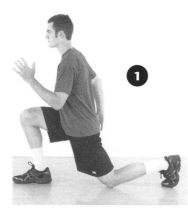

1

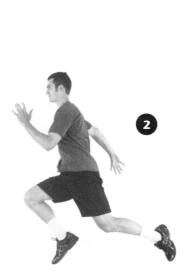

2

1–2 Keeping your back vertical, lower your body about 10 inches and explosively jump off of your front leg, springing into the air.

3 When landing, maintain the same lunge position. Do not allow the knee of your forward leg to extend in front of your foot.

Repeat, then switch sides.

3

BENEFIT

Develops overall power and explosiveness of the hip flexors and extensors.

Speed

Jump

STARTING POSITION: Stand in a split-squat position with your right foot and left arm forward. Keep your chest up.

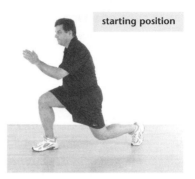

starting position

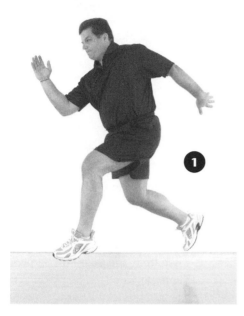

1 Jump and scissor your arms and legs at the same time so that your right arm comes forward with your left leg.

2 Upon landing, jump and scissor your legs back to your original starting position.

Repeat.

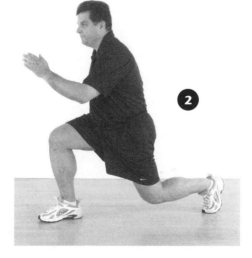

BENEFIT

Develops overall power and explosiveness, as well as dynamic flexibility, of the hip flexors and extensors.

lower-body plyos
split jumps with cycle

Speed

Jump

STARTING POSITION: Begin in a lunging position with your right leg forward, right knee and hip flexed and right foot flat on the ground. The left leg should be slightly flexed at the knee, with the ball of your left foot on the ground.

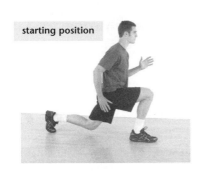

starting position

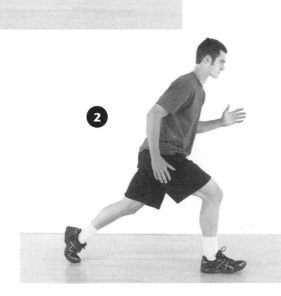

1

2

1–2 Explode off your right leg to jump straight up in the air. While in the air, pop your left heel to your butt and cycle your legs so that upon landing your left leg is in front and your right leg is in back.

Repeat single efforts, alternating legs.

BENEFIT

Develops overall quickness, as well as dynamic flexibility, of the quadriceps, hip flexors and hip extensors.

Speed

Jump

COD

STARTING POSITION: Stand in the athletic ready position, with knees slightly bent, back flat, and shoulders in front of hips.

starting position

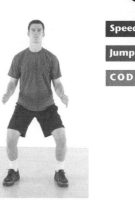

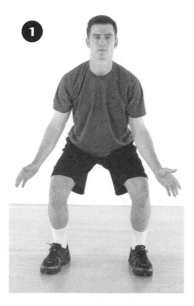

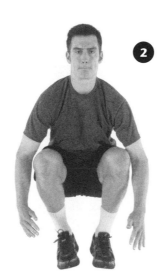

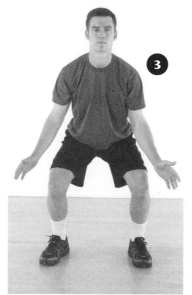

1 Quickly push your hips back while flexing your knees to lower into a quarter-squat.

2 Without pausing at the bottom of the squat, reverse direction and explosively jump straight up into the air, popping your knees up toward your chest.

3 When landing, make sure that you absorb the impact by pushing your hips back and flexing your knees.

Repeat single efforts for desired number of repetitions, or as a series of multiple-repetition jumps.

BENEFIT

Develops overall quickness, explosiveness of the hip flexors and dynamic flexibility of the hip extensors.

Speed

Jump

COD

STARTING POSITION: Stand with your feet hip-width apart and your arms at your sides. Lift your left foot so that it is not in contact with the ground.

starting position

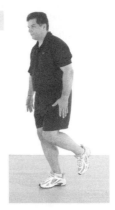

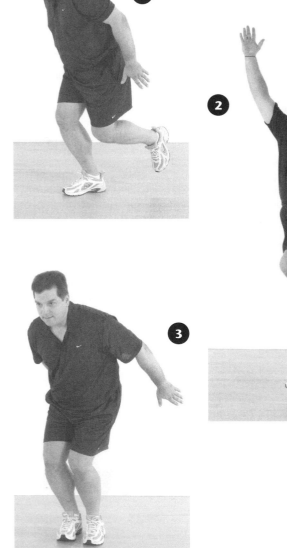

1 Keeping your weight on your right heel, quickly push your hips back while flexing your right knee to lower into a quarter-squat. As you do this, swing your arms backward.

2 Without pausing at the bottom of the squat, reverse direction explosively and jump straight up into the air.

3 Land on both feet.

Repeat single efforts, then switch sides.

BENEFIT

Develops overall quickness and deceleration ability, as well as dynamic balance of the lower leg muscles.

lower-body plyos
squat jumps (one leg)
level I

101

Speed

Jump

COD

STARTING POSITION: Stand with your feet hip-width apart and your hands behind your head. Lift your left foot so that it is not in contact with the ground.

starting position

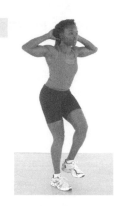

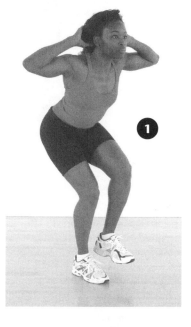

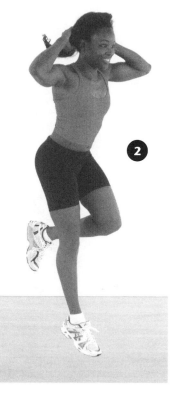

1 Pushing your hips back and flexing your right knee, lower into a quarter-squat. Pause in this position.

2 Without using your arms, jump as high as possible.

3 Land on your right foot, flexing the knee slightly to absorb landing impact.

Repeat single efforts, then switch sides.

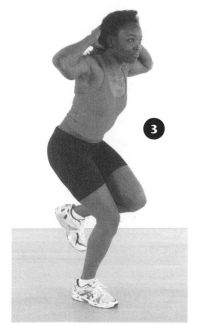

BENEFIT

Develops overall quickness and deceleration ability, as well as dynamic balance of the lower leg muscles.

STARTING POSITION: Stand with your feet hip-width apart and your arms at your sides. Face the direction of your jump.

starting position

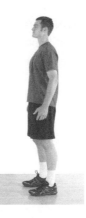

1

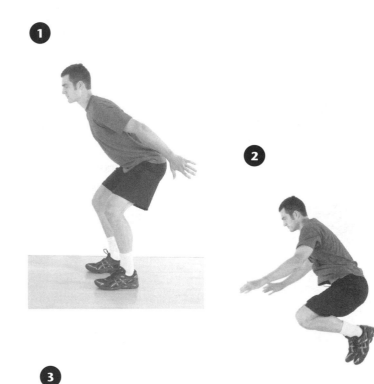

2

3

1 Quickly push your hips back and flex your knees into a quarter-squat. As you do this, swing your arms backward.

2 Without pausing, jump forward as you swing your arms forward.

3 When landing, make sure that you absorb the impact by pushing your hips back and flexing your knees.

Repeat single efforts or multiple-repetition jumps.

BENEFIT

Develops overall power and enhances the lower body's ability to decelerate.

standing lateral jump
level I

STARTING POSITION: Stand with your feet hip-width apart and your arms at your sides. Face the direction of your jump.

starting position

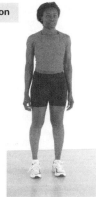

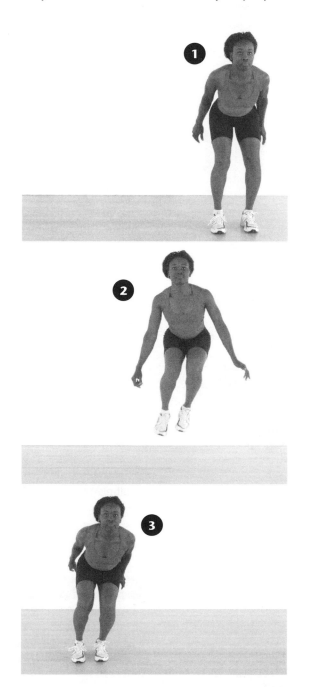

1 Quickly push your hips back and flex your knees into a quarter-squat. As you do this, swing your arms backward.

2 Without pausing, jump to the side as you swing your arms in the same direction.

3 When landing, make sure that you absorb the impact by pushing your hips back and flexing your knees.

Repeat single efforts or multiple-repetition jumps.

BENEFIT

Develops overall power and enhances the lower body's ability to decelerate and change direction explosively.

104
lower-body plyos
standing diagonal jump
level I

Jump

COD

STARTING POSITION: Stand with your feet hip-width apart and your arms at your sides. Face straight ahead.

starting position

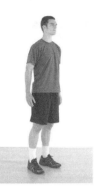

1

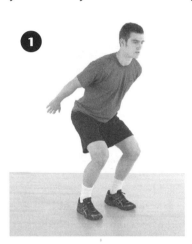

2

3

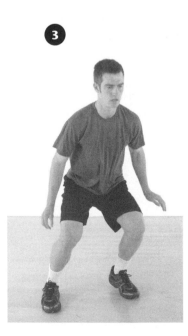

1 Quickly push your hips back and flex your knees into a quarter-squat. As you do this, swing your arms backward.

2 Without pausing, jump diagonally as you swing your arms in the same direction.

3 When landing, make sure that you absorb the impact by pushing your hips back and flexing your knees.

Repeat single efforts or multiple-repetition jumps.

BENEFIT

Develops overall power and enhances the lower body's ability to decelerate and change direction explosively.

Speed

Jump

STARTING POSITION: Stand with your feet hip-width apart, arms at your sides for balance. Lift your left foot so that it is not in contact with the ground.

starting position

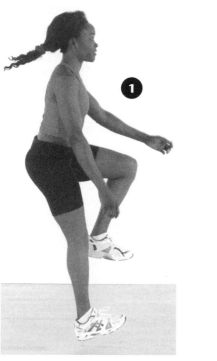

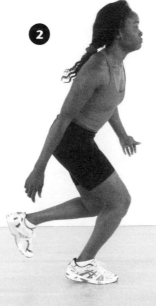

1 Push off with your right leg and jump forward, using a forceful swing of your left leg to increase the length of the jump but aiming primarily for height off each jump. Keep your body vertical and straight.

2 Land on the ball of the right foot and immediately take off again. Keep the foot touch-down time as short as possible.

Repeat, then switch legs.

BENEFIT

Develops overall power and explosiveness.

Jump

COD

STARTING POSITION: Stand with your feet hip-width apart and your arms at your sides. Face straight ahead.

starting position

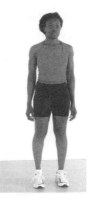

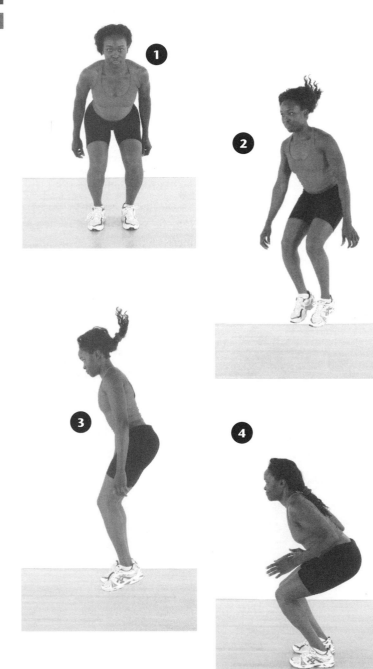

1 Quickly push your hips back and flex your knees into a quarter-squat. As you do this, swing your arms backward.

2–3 Without pausing, jump forward and rotate your trunk and hips to the right of your starting position.

4 When landing, make sure that you absorb the impact by pushing your hips back and flexing your knees.

Repeat, alternating between turns to your left then your right. Repeat single efforts or multiple-repetition jumps.

BENEFIT

Develops overall power and enhances body control, as well as an athlete's ability to change direction explosively.

ankle hops

Ankle hops may be done in place or in multiple directions.

STARTING POSITION: Stand with your feet hip-width apart, arms at your sides. Keep your knees slightly flexed and "soft" while performing ankle hops, but avoid using them to jump.

starting position

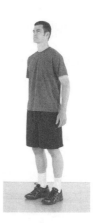

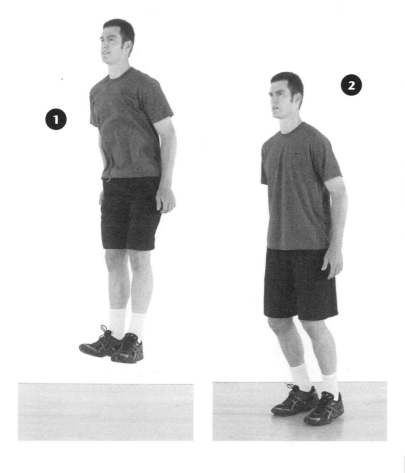

1 Quickly push your toes into the ground and explode up off the ground.

2 Land on the balls of your feet, "reloading" your ankles immediately by flexing your ankles into the flat-footed position.

Repeat.

BENEFIT

Conditions and develops the dynamic balance of the muscles in the lower leg.

Jump

COD

Multiple hops may be done in place or in multiple directions.

STARTING POSITION: Stand with your feet hip-width apart and your arms at your sides.

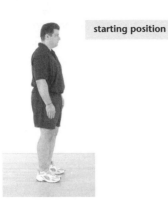
starting position

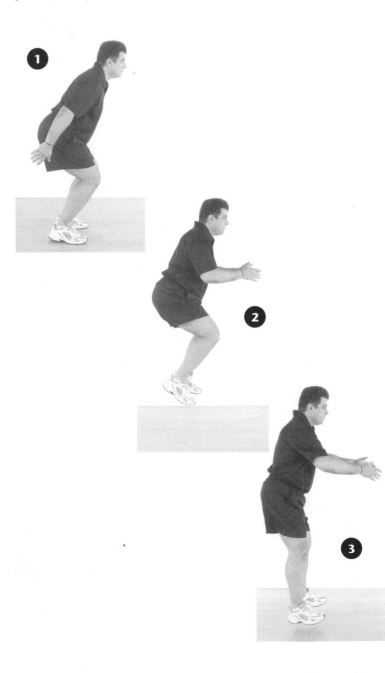

1 Quickly push your hips back and flex your knees into a quarter-squat. As you do this, swing your arms backward.

2 Without pausing, jump forward as you swing your arms forward. Emphasize proper technique and getting off the ground quickly.

3 Upon landing, absorb the impact by pushing your hips back and flexing your knees, and immediately repeat, jumping forward again.

Repeat multiple jumps for desired number of repetitions.

BENEFIT

Conditions and develops your legs' ability to decelerate during sprinting or jumping.

Speed

Jump

COD

STARTING POSITION: Stand with your feet about shoulder-width apart and your knees slightly bent, arms at your sides.

starting position

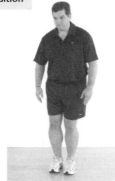

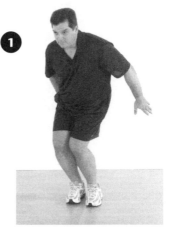

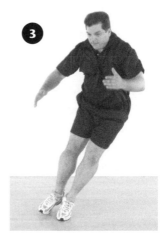

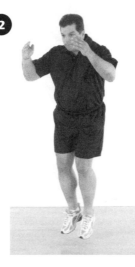

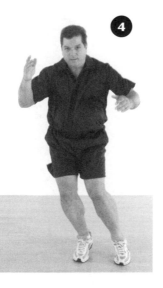

1–2 Flexing your knees to quickly drop your body 10 to 12 inches, rapidly explode upward, forward and to the side. Swing your arms forcefully upward.

3–4 Upon landing, immediately jump forward diagonally in the opposite direction.

Repeat.

BENEFIT

Develops overall power and enhances body control, as well as an athlete's ability to decelerate and change direction explosively.

target hops

level I

STARTING POSITION: Set up 4 quadrants adjacent to each other by creating a cross using masking tape. Stand with your feet together and your body facing the first quadrant. (For more precise footwork, you may also arrange small pieces of tape in a pattern of your choice.)

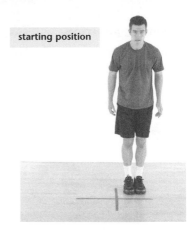

starting position

1 Hop forward using both feet and land in the first quadrant.

2 Immediately hop and land in the quadrant to the side.

3 Then jump backward to land in the quadrant behind you.

4 Finish by jumping to your right to land in the final quadrant.

Repeat, switching directions.

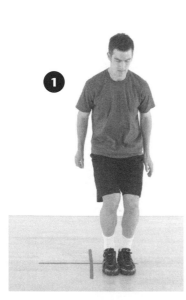

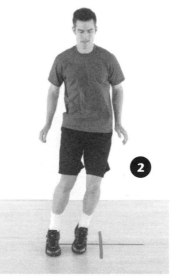

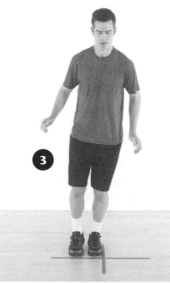

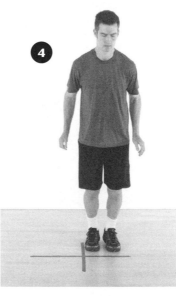

BENEFIT

Develops overall power and enhances body control, as well as an athlete's ability to decelerate and change direction explosively.

Jump

COD

STARTING POSITION: Set up 4 quadrants adjacent to each other by creating a cross using masking tape. Stand in one quadrant on one foot, with the other foot held free behind your body. (For more precise footwork, you may also arrange small pieces of tape in a pattern of your choice.)

starting position

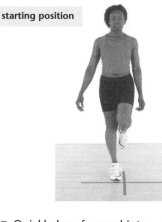

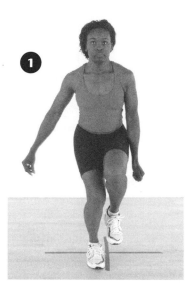

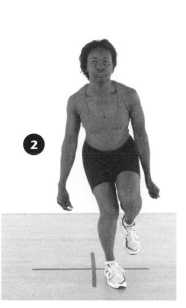

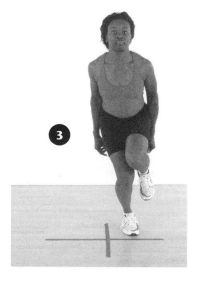

1 Quickly hop forward into the first quadrant.

2 Immediately upon landing, hop to the next quadrant.

3 Continue hopping back and forth in your desired pattern, spending as little time as possible on the ground upon landing each hop.

Repeat, then switch sides.

BENEFIT

Enhances dynamic stability of the lower leg.

lower-body plyos

slalom hops (one leg)

level I

STARTING POSITION: Stand on one foot with your other foot held free behind your body.

starting position

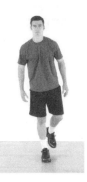

1–2 Flexing your knee to quickly drop your body 10 to 12 inches, rapidly explode upward, forward and to the side. Swing your arms forcefully upward.

3 Land on the same leg and immediately repeat the exercise with that leg, jumping forward but in the opposite direction in a zig-zag pattern. Strive for maximum distance on each hop.

Repeat for the desired number of repetitions or for a specific time or distance. Switch sides.

BENEFIT

Enhances dynamic stability of the lower leg.

Arrange a series of cones or hurdles two to three feet apart, for as many jumps as you desire. You can mix and match hurdles of varying heights to add some variety to this exercise.

STARTING POSITION: Stand in a semi-squat position 1 to 2 feet away from the first cone. Feet should be slightly wider than hip-width apart.

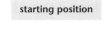
starting position

Speed

Jump

COD

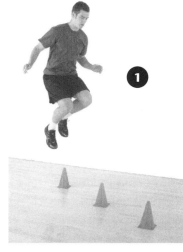

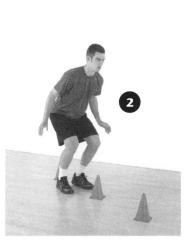

1–2 Driving your arms up and taking off from both feet, jump over the cone. The movement should come from your hips and knees; keep your body vertical and straight. Land on the balls of your feet and . . .

3–4 . . . quickly jump over the next cone. Use the double-arm swing to maintain balance and gain height.

Repeat.

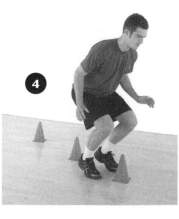

BENEFIT

Conditions and develops your legs' ability to decelerate during sprinting or jumping.

STARTING POSITION: Set up 2 markers about 4 feet apart. Stand on your left leg on the left edge of the designated space, keeping your right leg behind you and your right toes on the ground for balance.

starting position

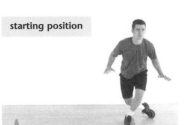

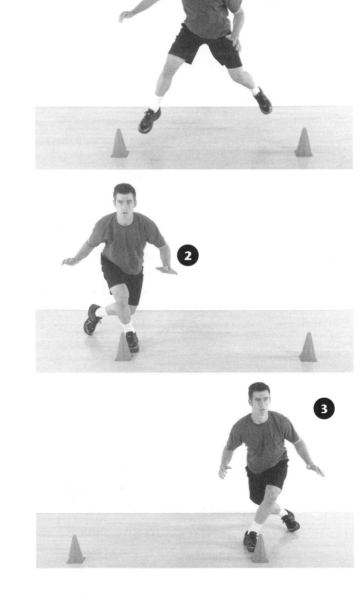

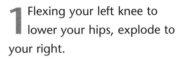

1 Flexing your left knee to lower your hips, explode to your right.

2 Land on your right foot, bending your right knee to absorb your landing impact and bringing your left leg behind your right foot to counter-balance as you decelerate.

3 Immediately reverse direction, leaping back onto your left foot.

Repeat.

BENEFIT

Develops quick and explosive change of direction as well as dynamic stability of the entire leg.

alternating straddle hops   *level I*

This exercise can also be done using a step.

STARTING POSITION: Stand to the right side of a box and place your left foot on top of the box.

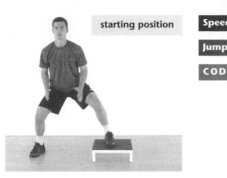

starting position

Speed

Jump

COD

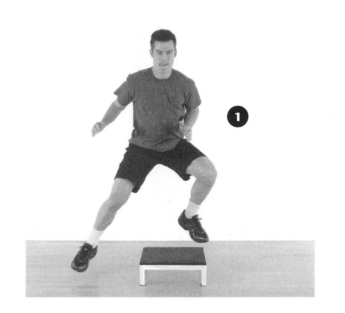

1 Using the left leg only, push off the box and explode vertically as high as possible. Drive the arms forward and up for maximum height.

2 Land on the other side of the box with your opposite foot on the box.

Immediately repeat, alternating sides.

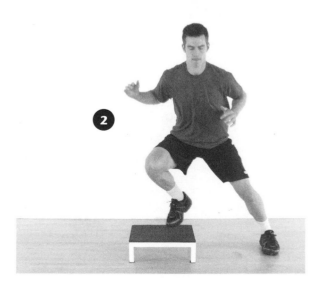

BENEFIT

Develops overall power and explosiveness, as well as dynamic flexibility of the hip adductors.

lower-body plyos

box jumps

Speed

Jump

COD

This can also be done with several boxes instead of one. The height of the box may vary, but should be in the region of 12 to 30 inches.

STARTING POSITION: Stand with your feet shoulder-width apart facing a 12-inch box. Contract your abdominal muscles to stabilize your trunk and spine.

starting position

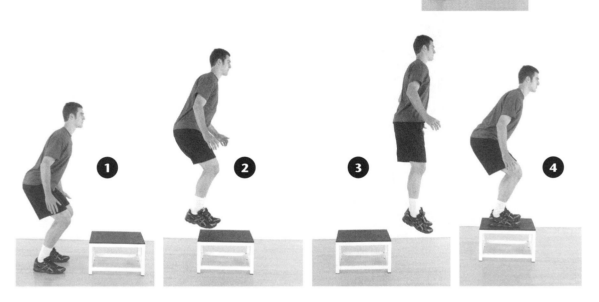

1–2 Quickly drop down into a squatting position and immediately jump onto the box, landing softly on the balls of your feet in a squat position.

3 Jump off the box onto the ground, landing softly on the balls of your feet in a squat position.

4 Jump back onto the box, keeping the feet touch-down time on the ground as short as possible.

Repeat for one to three sets, allowing for full recovery between each set.

BENEFIT

Develops overall power and explosiveness, and enhances the lower body's ability to decelerate.

STARTING POSITION: Stand on a box with your arms at your sides. Contract your abdominal muscles to stabilize your trunk and spine.

starting position

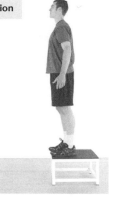

Speed

Jump

COD

1 Step—don't jump—off of the bench with your right foot.

2 As soon as you land, explode vertically as high as you can. Try to minimize ground-contact time—don't sink down into a deep squat before jumping up.

Repeat, alternating legs.

1

2

BENEFIT

Develops overall power and explosiveness, and enhances the lower body's ability to decelerate.

box jump-ups

Speed
Jump
COD

This exercise can also be done using a weight bench.

STARTING POSITION: Stand directly in front of a box with your right foot firmly placed on top of the box and your left foot on the floor. Your left arm should be forward, elbow bent about 90 degrees.

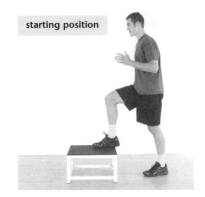

starting position

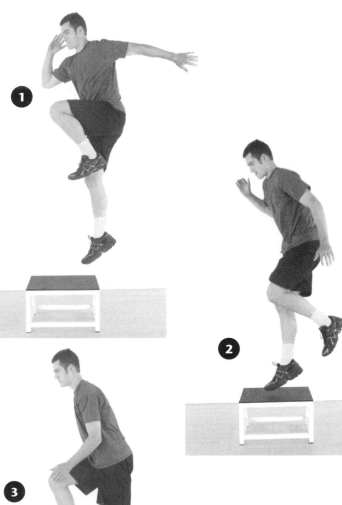

1 Press up onto the box with your right foot and explode your left knee up toward the ceiling, causing both feet to lift off the box. Your right arm should come forward, as it would when sprinting.

2–3 Land with your right foot back on the box and your left foot on the floor, your arms reversing directions.

Repeat, then switch legs.

BENEFIT

Develops the power and explosiveness of each hip extensor and extensor.

upper-body plyos
push-ups (off the wall)
level 1

119

STARTING POSITION: Stand facing a wall a little more than arm's length away and place your hands on the wall, arms fully extended.

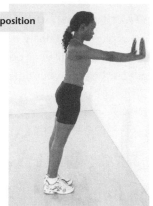

starting position

Push-Pull

1

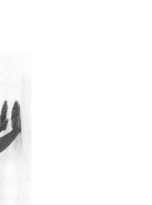

1 Lean from your ankles and "fall" toward the wall. "Catch" yourself by placing your hands flat on the wall, bending your elbows and bringing your chest toward the wall.

2

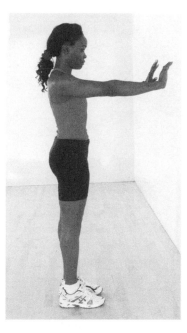

2 Reverse direction explosively, pushing off the wall with a maximal extension of the arms and driving your body away from the wall.

Repeat.

BENEFIT

Develops overall power and explosiveness of the upper body.

Push-Pull

STARTING POSITION: From standing, place your hands on either side of a stability ball. Without moving your feet, roll the ball forward until your body forms a straight line from the top of your head to your heels.

starting position

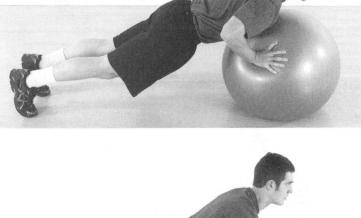

1 Bend your elbows out to the sides to lower your chest to the ball. Maintain the straight line from head to heels.

2 Press through the heels, pads and fingers of your hands to push back up to starting position.

Repeat.

VARIATIONS

Level II: You can do this exercise without the ball. Lower your chest toward the floor then explode upward, lifting your body off the floor. Keep your elbows bent and wrists prepared to catch the landing and explode immediately into the next push-up.

Level I: Rather than start on your hands and the balls of your feet, rest your knees on the ground, making sure to keep your back straight.

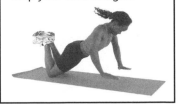

BENEFIT

Develops overall power and explosiveness of the upper body.

push-press

STARTING POSITION: Hold a barbell with an overhand grip, hands slightly wider than shoulder width. Position the bar chest high, keeping your back straight and retracting your head back.

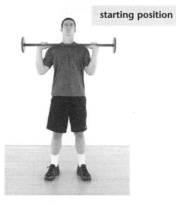

starting position

Speed

Jump

COD

Push-Pull

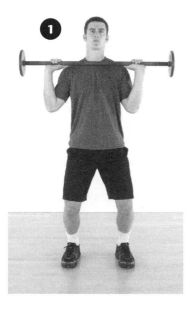

1 Dip your body by bending your knees, hips and ankles slightly.

2 Explosively drive upward with your legs, driving the barbell up off your shoulders and vigorously extending your arms overhead.

Return to starting position and repeat.

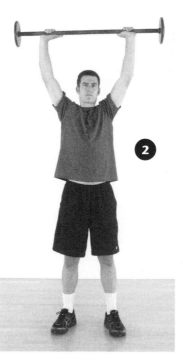

BENEFIT
Develops overall power and explosiveness of the upper body.

Speed

Jump

COD

Push-Pull

STARTING POSITION: Stand over a barbell with the balls of your feet positioned slightly wider than hip-width apart under the bar. Squat down and grip the bar with an overhand grip, hands slightly wider than shoulder width. Position your shoulders over the bar with your back arched tightly. Keep your arms straight with your elbows pointed along the bar.

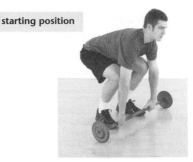
starting position

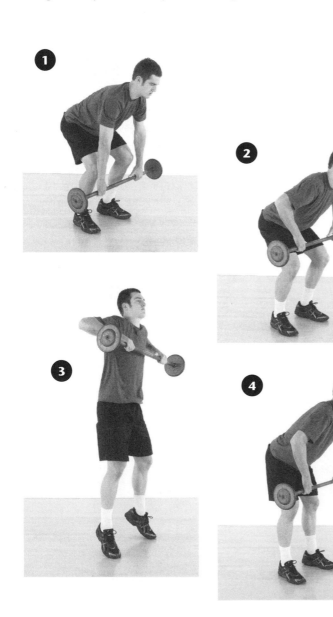

1 Extend your hips and knees to pull the bar up off the floor.

2–3 As the bar reaches your knees, vigorously shrug your shoulders; while keeping the barbell close to your thighs, simultaneously jump upward, extending your body. Flex your elbows out to the sides while pulling the bar up to neck height.

4 Bend your knees slightly and lower the barbell to mid-thigh position. Slowly lower the bar with your lower back taut and your trunk close to vertical.

Repeat.

BENEFIT

Develops overall power and explosiveness.

Speed

Jump

COD

Push-Pull

This exercise is typically performed using rubber weightlifting plates on a weightlifting platform, in which case you may drop the bar from the completed position. This technique reduces the stress or fatigue involved in lowering the bar as prescribed.

STARTING POSITION: From standing, hold a barbell with an overhand grip slightly wider than shoulder width. Bend your knees and hips so the barbell touches mid-thigh. Position your shoulders over the bar with your back arched. Keep your arms straight with your elbows pointed along the bar.

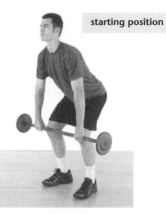

starting position

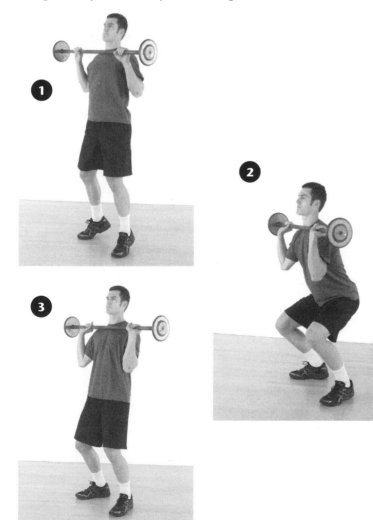

1 Jump upward, extending your body. Simultaneously shrug your shoulders and pull the barbell upward with your arms, allowing your elbows to flex out to the sides, keeping the bar close to your body. Aggressively pull your body under the bar, rotating your elbows around the bar.

2 Catch the bar on your shoulders while moving into a squat position.

3 Upon hitting the bottom of the squat, stand up immediately.

Repeat.

BENEFIT

Develops overall power and explosiveness of the whole body.

tricep press pass

This is an ideal exercise for soccer players as it exactly mimics the inbound throw in soccer. This can also be done with a partner.

Push-Pull

STARTING POSITION: Stand opposite a wall with one foot slightly in front of the other, holding a medicine ball in both hands with your arms fully extended overhead.

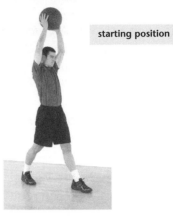

starting position

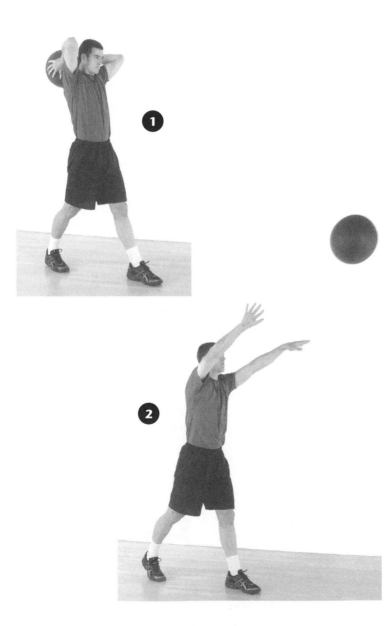

1 Flex both elbows, bringing the ball back behind your head.

2 Quickly reverse direction, explosively extending the elbows and releasing the ball forward as the arms fully extend overhead.

Repeat.

BENEFIT

Focuses on the triceps while stimulating all of the anterior muscles of the trunk.

STARTING POSITION: Stand with your feet wider than hip width and hold a medicine ball above your head

starting position

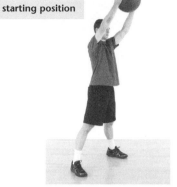

Jump

Push-Pull

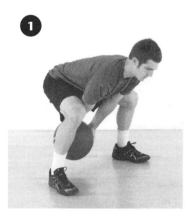

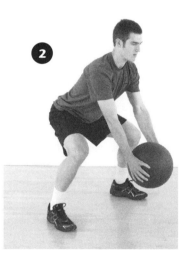

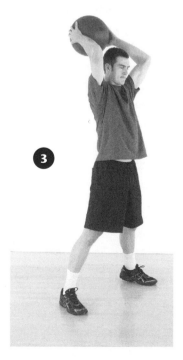

1 Shift your hips down and back as if squatting, keeping your back straight, and allow the medicine ball to swing back in-between your legs.

2–3 Reverse the motion by extending your hips, knees and ankles and allowing your shoulders and medicine ball to come up high overhead.

Repeat.

BENEFIT

Develops overall explosiveness and power through the hips and trunk.

squat throws

Jump

Push-Pull

STARTING POSITION: Stand with your feet hip-width apart and your knees slightly bent. Hold a medicine ball at chest level.

starting position

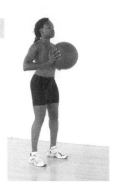

1 Squat down so that your thighs are parallel to the floor, then . . .

2 . . . quickly explode up and jump as high as you can while pressing the ball up. You should reach full extension with your arms when you are at the peak of your jump. Push the ball as high as possible into the air. Try to minimize the time spent in the squatted position—it should be a quick squat and jump.

Repeat.

BENEFIT

Develops overall explosiveness and power through the hips, trunk and shoulders.

This can also be done with a partner, who allows the ball to come to his/her chest before passing it back to you.

STARTING POSITION: Stand opposite a wall with your feet hip-width apart and knees slightly bent. Hold the medicine ball with both hands at chest level, your elbows pointing out.

starting position

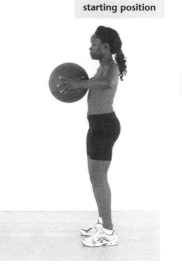

Push-
Pull

1 Explosively throw the medicine ball against the wall, pushing it off your chest and ending with your arms straight in front of you. Avoid snapping your elbows.

Anticipate the catch and return the ball as quickly as you can. Repeat.

BENEFIT

Develops overall explosiveness and power through the trunk, chest and shoulders.

Push-Pull

This can also be done with a partner.

STARTING POSITION: Stand opposite a wall with your feet hip-width apart and knees slightly bent. Hold a medicine ball above your head, arms fully extended.

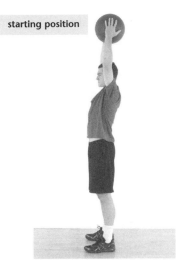

starting position

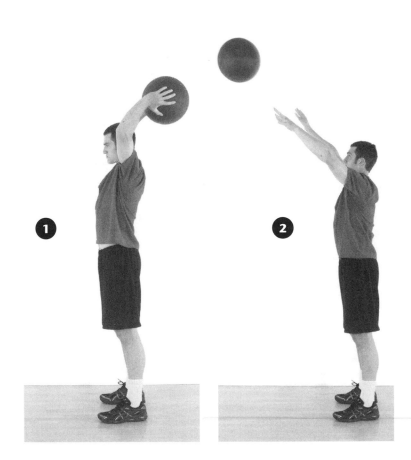

1 With your arms still extended, stretch your arms backward to move the ball behind your head. Try not to arch your lower back too much.

2 Throw the ball against the wall, releasing it just behind or above your head.

Anticipate the catch and return the ball as quickly as you can. Repeat.

BENEFIT

Develops overall explosiveness and power through the trunk and chest.

This drill requires a partner.

STARTING POSITION: Lie with your back on a stability ball with knees bent; have your partner stand a distance away. Hold a medicine ball directly over your chest with your arms extended.

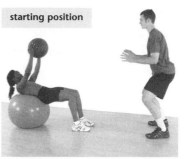

starting position

Push-Pull

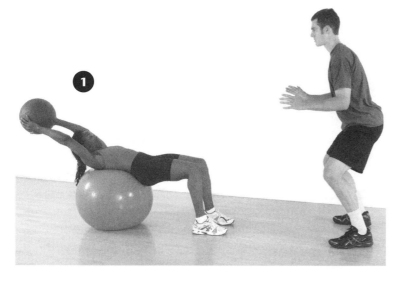

1 With your arms still extended, lower the ball behind your head as far as you can without dropping it on the floor.

2 Throw the ball forward toward your feet, releasing it when your arms are straight over your chest and abdomen.

Have your partner pass the ball back to you and repeat.

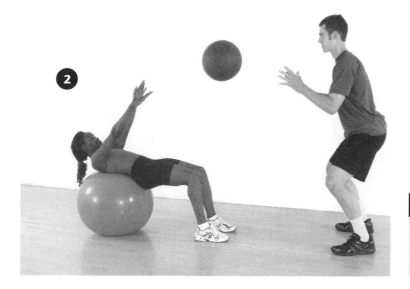

BENEFIT

Develops overall explosiveness and power through the trunk, chest and back.

STARTING POSITION: Sit on the floor with your legs partially extended and your feet flat on the floor. Hold a medicine ball in front of your chest with your arms extended, keeping your elbows slightly flexed.

starting position

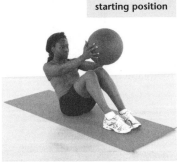

Rotate

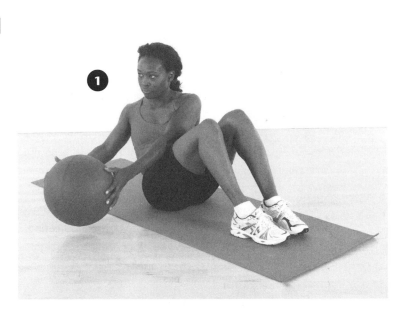

1 Rotate to your right and lightly tap the medicine ball on the floor to your right.

2 Immediately and quickly reverse direction, rotating to your left and lightly tap the medicine ball on the floor to your left.

Repeat.

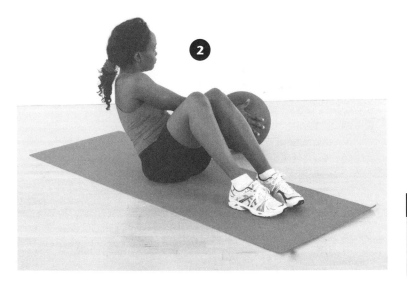

BENEFIT

Develops explosiveness and power through the trunk.

This drill requires a partner.

STARTING POSITION: Stand with your feet hip-width apart. Hold a medicine ball out at chest level with your arms extended but your elbows slightly flexed. Your partner stands a distance away to your right.

starting position

Rotate

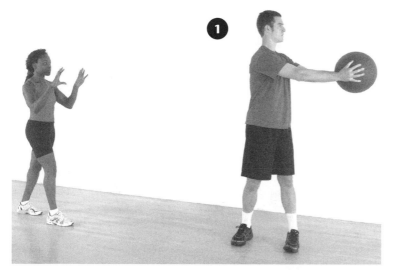

1 Rotate toward your left.

2 Quickly reverse direction, rotating explosively to your right and tossing the ball to your partner.

Repeat, then switch sides.

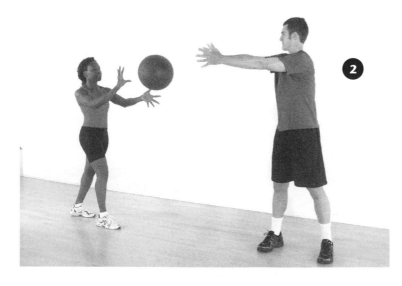

BENEFIT

Enhances rotational power of the trunk.

This drill requires a partner.

STARTING POSITION: Stand with your feet together. Hold the medicine ball at hip level. Your partner stands a distance away to your right.

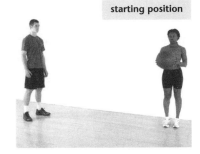

starting position

Rotate

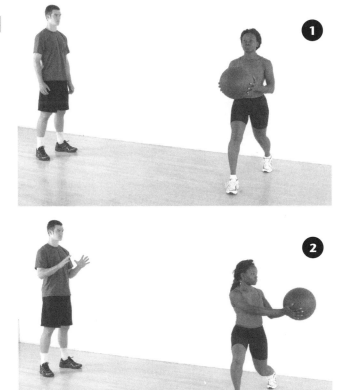

1–2 Step back with your left foot into a lunge position and rotate toward the left. Extend your arms but keep your elbows slightly flexed.

3 Quickly reverse direction, rotating explosively to your right and tossing the ball to your partner.

Repeat, then switch sides.

BENEFIT

Improves balance and coordination, as well as increases the stretch of the hip flexors.

upper-body plyos
rotating pass on ball
level III

133

This drill requires a partner.

STARTING POSITION: Lie on your back on a stability ball. Your feet should be wide and flat on the floor, with your knees bent 90 degrees. Hold a medicine ball out in front of your chest with your arms extended but your elbows slightly flexed. Your partner stands a distance away to your left.

starting position

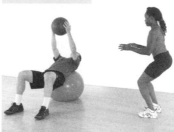

Rotate

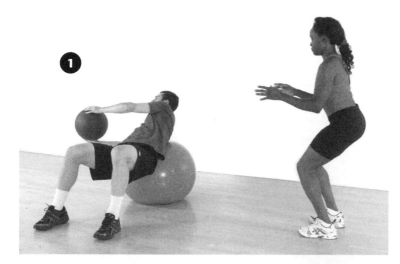

1 Roll on the ball to your right, bringing the medicine ball to your right with your arms extended.

2 Quickly reverse direction and rotate toward your left, tossing the ball to your partner. Stay as evenly balanced on the stability ball as possible.

Repeat, alternating sides.

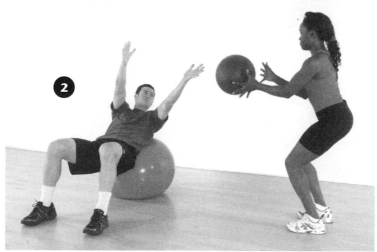

BENEFIT

Develops rotational power through the hips and trunk.

medicine ball slams

level I

Jump

Push-
Pull

STARTING POSITION: Stand with your feet parallel and knees slightly bent. Hold a medicine ball at chest level.

starting position

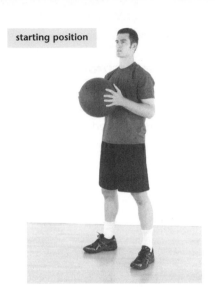

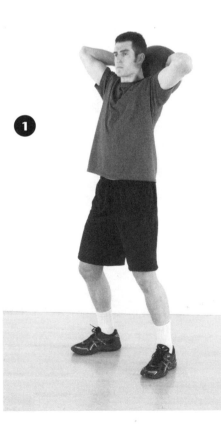

1 Pull the medicine ball back behind your head and forcefully throw the ball down on the ground as hard as possible.

Catch the ball on the bounce from the ground and repeat.

BENEFIT

Develops overall explosiveness and power through the trunk.

This can also be done with a partner.

STARTING POSITION: Stand facing a wall with your feet hip-width apart and your knees slightly bent. Hold the medicine ball in your left hand, with the back of your hand against the front of your left shoulder.

starting position

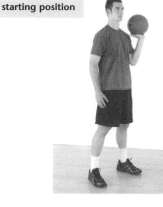

Push-
Pull

1 Shot-put the ball as force-fully as possible against the wall; avoid snapping your elbow.

2 Catch the ball on the rebound.

Repeat, alternating sides.

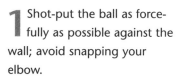

BENEFIT

Develops explosiveness and power through the chest, shoulders and arms.

rotational slams

This can also be done with a partner.

STARTING POSITION: Stand with a wall to your right. Place your feet hip-width apart, with your left foot approximately one foot in front of the right. Hold the medicine ball in front of you, keeping your arms slightly bent.

starting position

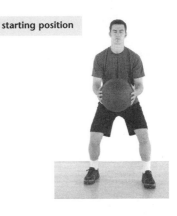

Rotate

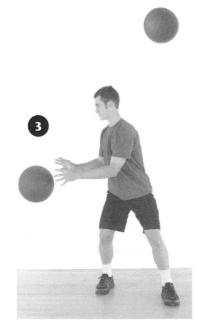

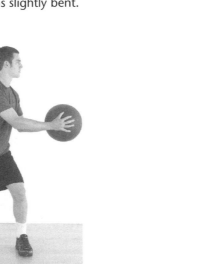

1–2 Rotate your trunk to the left, swinging the ball past your left hip. Quickly and forcefully rotate your torso from left to right to toss the ball against the wall.

3 Catch the ball on the rebound.

Repeat.

BENEFIT

Develops rotational power through the hips and trunk.

This can also be done with a partner.

STARTING POSITION: Stand facing a wall with your feet wider than hip-width apart, knees bent. Let your arms hang down with the medicine ball held in front of your hips.

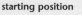
starting position

Jump

Push-Pull

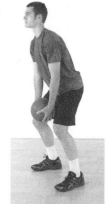

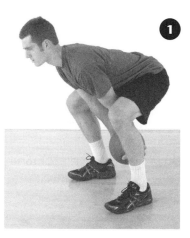

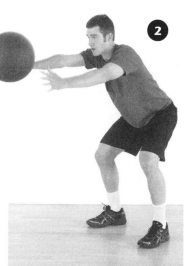

1 Shift your hips down and back as if squatting while maintaining a straight back, and allow the medicine ball to swing back in-between your legs.

2 Reverse the motion by extending your hips, knees and ankles and tossing the ball forward against the wall.

3 Catch the ball on the rebound.

Repeat.

BENEFIT

Develops overall power and explosiveness through the hips and trunk.

Speed

Push-Pull

This drill requires enough space for you to be able to throw the medicine ball in front of you and actually sprint about 10 yards.

STARTING POSITION: Stand with your feet slightly wider than hip-width apart and your knees slightly bent. Bend at the waist and step back with your left foot, keeping both knees and ankles flexed. Hold the medicine ball at face level.

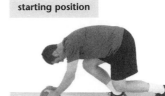

starting position

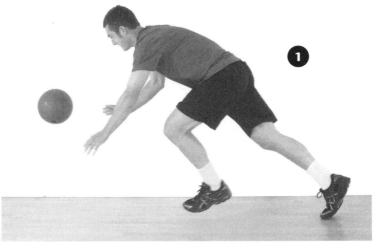

1 Quickly explode up and press the ball straight out as far and as fast as you can.

2 As you press the ball forward, explode with either leg so that you sprint forward a couple of steps.

Repeat.

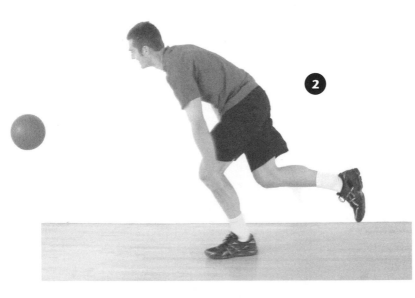

BENEFIT

Develops explosiveness and power through the hips and trunk.

This drill can also be done with a partner standing approximately 10 to 15 yards behind you.

STARTING POSITION: Stand 10 to 15 yards in front of a high wall with your feet slightly wider than hip-width apart and knees bent. Hold the ball in front of you.

starting position

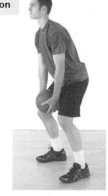

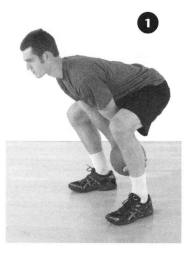

1 Lower your body into a semi-squat position.

2 Explode up, extending your entire body and throwing the medicine ball up and over your body. The goal is to throw the ball behind you as far as you can and generating most of the power from your legs.

Repeat.

BENEFIT

Develops explosiveness and power through the hips and trunk.

140

upper-body plyos
push "over the top"
level II

Push-
Pull

This can also be done using a medicine ball or BOSU.

STARTING POSITION: Start in a prone push-up position with your feet wide, your arms extended, and your left hand on the step.

starting position

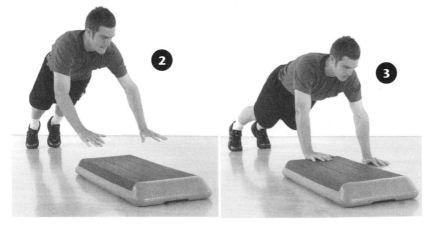

1 Quickly bend your elbows, dropping your chest toward the floor, and then . . .

2–3 . . . explode upward with a maximal extension of your arms and chest, lifting your body over the step and placing your right hand on the step and your left hand on the floor.

4 Descend your chest toward the floor quickly and explode upward in the opposite direction, moving into the next repetition without pausing between reps.

Repeat, alternating sides.

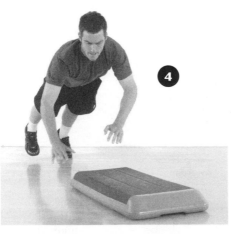

BENEFIT

Develops explosiveness and power through the hips and trunk.

upper-body plyos
upper-body forward hops
level III

141

If using a towel, this should be done on a wooden floor.

STARTING POSITION: Start in a prone, "on-knees" push-up position, keeping your arms extended and your knees together on the towel or Ab-Dolly.

starting position

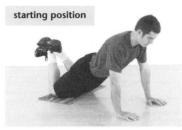

Push-Pull

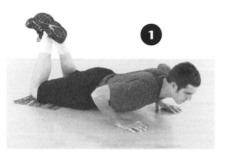

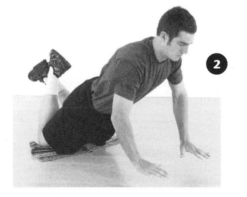

1–2 Quickly bend your elbows, dropping your chest toward the floor, and then explode upward with a maximal extension of the arms and chest, lifting your body forward as you roll forward.

3 As you land on both hands, descend your chest toward the floor quickly and explode upward again without pausing between reps.

Repeat.

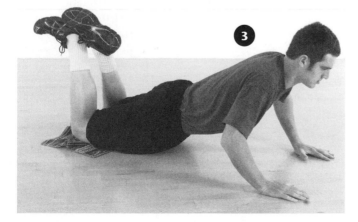

BENEFIT
Develops power and quickness through the anterior chain of the upper body.

index

about the author

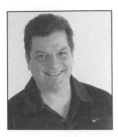

NEAL PIRE, MA, FACSM, is the director at Sports Training Academy in Ridgewood, New Jersey. A certified strength and conditioning specialist for over 27 years, Neal has been listed as one of the top ten fitness directors and educators in the nation by the American Council on Exercise. He also serves on the executive council for the Committee on Certification and Registry Board for the American College of Sports Medicine.

Neal has worked extensively with athletes at all levels, from developmental Pee-Wee soccer players to Olympic figure skaters to NFL pro football players. He has served on the sports medicine team for USA Track and Field and the New York City Marathon, and is currently a strength and conditioning specialist for USA Swimming's Sports Medicine and Science Network.

about the photographer

ANDY MOGG is a well-known and much-published photographer. Born in England in 1954, he worked as a consultant, then writer and photographer. At 17, he moved from London to Belgium, traveling and working his way through Europe; he settled in the United States 20 years ago. He now runs a thriving photography studio in Oakland, California. For more information, visit his website at www.dancingimages.com.

acknowledgments

From the author: I thank my daughters Taryn and Nikki for helping to keep me grounded and maintain clear priorities. I also acknowledge Tom Burke and Sue Higgins, among my many mentors over the years, for feeding my hunger for knowledge and understanding of both the science and art of training and conditioning. To Lew Maharam and Liz Neporent, for driving me to excellence and professional growth. And very special thanks to you who have touched my heart, inspiring and sharing my passion and desire to positively impact the world, if only one person at a time. &

From the publisher: The publisher would like to thank Benita Smolny and Maria Cruz at the Oakland YMCA for the use of the facilities. Coach Curtis Taylor of Laney College generously loaned us the plyometrics boxes used in the shoot. And most of all, thank you to fitness models Samuel Denton-Schneider and Vanessa Alvarez for participating in this project.